The Complete Book of Family Homeopathic Medicine

Maesimund B. Panos, M.D.
Jane Heimlich

Rhus Tox - poison ivy plant.

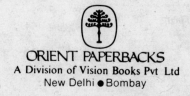

ORIENT PAPERBACKS
A Division of Vision Books Pvt Ltd
New Delhi • Bombay

ISBN 81-222-0081-8
First Indian Edition 1983

The Complete Book of Family Homeopathic Medicine
(published originally as *Homeopathic Medicine at Home*)

© Mae simund B. Panos M.D.,
   Jane Heimlich

Cover design by Vision Studio

Published in arrangement with J.P. Tarcher, Inc.,/Houghton Mifflin Co., 2, Park Street, Boston, Mass., 02108 U.S.A.

Published by
Orient Paperbacks
(A Division of Vision Books Pvt. Ltd.)
Madarsa Road, Kashmere Gate, Delhi-110 006

Printed in India
at Gopsons Paper Pvt. Ltd.,
Noida, U.P.

Cover Printed at
Ravindra Printing Press, Delhi-110 006.

Foreword

WOULD you like to know how to use inexpensive, effective, natural remedies that have no side effects? If so, *Homeopathic Medicine at Home* is the book for you.

Saturated in homeopathy by heredity and marriage (both her father and deceased husband were homeopaths), training (after she finished Ohio State College of Medicine, an internship, and residency, she was assistant to a homeopath), and her own private practice, Dr. Maesimund B. Panos is superbly qualified to teach all of us about homeopathy.

And, as overwhelming numbers of people lose faith in modern medicine, this is the right era for us to learn about this time-honored method of healing, whose preparations are obtained from animal, vegetable, and mineral sources. As the image of penicillin is tarnished by the reality of allergic reactions, why not examine *Belladonna* (a homeopathic—and, therefore, safe—remedy prepared from deadly nightshade) as an appropriate treatment for strep throat. As concerned parents reject phenobarbitol for their colicky infant, why not try *Bryonia*. As obstetrics and pediatrics are rocked by the scandals of thalidomide and its descendants, why not reduce morning sickness with *Colchicum*. As the evidence of dangers such as gastrointestinal bleeding from aspirin mounts, why not choose *Gelsemium* to get rid of your tension headache. And, rather than relying on habitforming laxatives, why not use *Nux* to break the habit.

Coauthor Jane Heimlich's pen provides plenty of highly literate, easily readable information for safely carrying out much of the homeopathic first-aid treatment in your own home.

In my medical education, the total field of homeopathy was presented in less than ten minutes. The attitude was condescending at best and, more accurately, derogatory. Because I have learned precious little about homeopathy in the intervening years, I was delighted when Jane Heimlich asked me to write a foreword to this important book. I wish that all doctors—and especially medical students—would read it; those who do will certainly have a head start on their colleagues for the 1980s. However, since most will not, we must be grateful to Maesimund Panos and Jane Heimlich for giving every responsible and concerned person a splendid opportunity to learn, easily and usefully, about this valuable alternative healing method.

Robert S. Mendelsohn, M.D.,
author of *Confessions of a Medical Heretic*

Note

The book indicates 2 tablets as dosage in all cases. But since pills and not tablets are more in use in India the user is advised to substitute 4-5 pills in place of 2 tablets.

Contents

Foreword — 3

What This Book Will Do for You — 9

1. **What is Homeopathy?** — 11
   Principles of Homeopathy / 12
   A Comparison of Homeopathy and Standard Medicine (Allopathy / 15
   Homeopathy and Naturopathy / 16
   Homeopathy and Herbalism / 16
   Homeopathy Suppressed in America / 17
   Homeopathy: the Alternative of the Future / 18

2. **A Homeopathic Physician At Work** — 20
   Taking the Case / 20
   The Making of A Homeopath / 23
   Homeopathy Versus Allopathy: A Practical View / 23
   The Satisfaction of Homeopathy / 25

3. **Your Home Remedy Kit** — 27
   The Homeopathic Household Kit / 28
   Observation: The Key to Prescribing / 34
   The Combination Game / 36

4. **What to Do For Accidents?** — 38
   Bruises (Contusions) / 38
   Sprains / 40
   Strains / 42
   Wounds / 42
   Insect Stings and Bites / 45
   Sports Injuries / 44
   Quick Reference Chart / 50

5. **In Case of Emergency** — 58
   Bleeding / 58
   Obstruction to Breathing / 59

Shock / 61
Fainting / 61
Poisoning / 62
Eye Injuries / 62
Fever / 63
Sunstroke / 65
Heat Prostration / 65
Dental Work / 66
Surgery / 67
Quick Reference Chart / 68

6. **How to Prevent and Treat Colds, Coughs and Earaches**   73

Colds / 73
Flu / 76
Coughs / 77
Earaches / 78
Quick Reference Chart / 79

7. **Remedies for Stomach and Bowel Problems**   88

Indigestion / 88
Nausea and Vomiting / 89
Gas / 90
Constipation / 91
Diarrhea / 92
Hemorrhoids (Piles) / 94
Quick Reference Chart / 96

8. **A Happier Baby with Homeopathic Care**   102

Poor Sleeping Habits / 103
Allergies / 104
Colds / 104
Earaches / 106
Colic / 107
Diarrhea / 108
Vomiting / 108
Diaper Rash / 109
Teething / 109
Quick Reference Chart / 111

9. **Your Growing Child**   116

The Toddler / 116
Poisoning / 116
Choking / 117
Falls and Bruises / 118
Burns / 119

Earaches / 120
Fever / 121
Croup / 121

The School Age Child / 122

Colds / 122
Tonsilitis / 123
Measles (Seven-Day Measles) / 124
Rubella (German Measles) / 125
Chicken Pox / 125
Mumps / 125
Scarlet Fever / 126
Warts / 126
Enuresis (Bed-Wetting) / 127
Fears and Anxieties / 129

The Adolescent / 129

Menstruation / 130
Acne / 131
Mononucleosis / 133
Emotions / 134
Quick Reference Chart / 136

10. **What Homeopathy can Do for Women** 145

Your Headache: Fast and Safe Relief / 145
Pregnancy; Morning Sickness / 147
Varicose Veins / 148
Urinary Problems / 148
Constipation / 149
Hemorrhoids / 149
Indigestion / 149
Insomnia / 150
Labor / 150
Postpartum Blues / 151
Breast-Feeding / 152
Menopause / 153
The Estrogen Question / 153
Quick Reference Chart / 155

11. **Keeping Your Pets Healthy** 161

Appendix A : Remedies and their Abbreviations / 165
Appendix B : Mini-Repertory / 167
Appendix C : Materia Medica / 172
Appendix D : Consumer's Guide to Homeopathic Medicine / 183

What This Book Will Do for You

As evidenced by the proliferating volume of books and magazines on health subjects, an increasing number of people want to be more self-sufficient in this area. You, too, may share this desire. With rising medical costs, you don't want to run to the doctor for every little thing. With a constant stream of reports appearing in the press about the dangers of commonly prescribed drugs, you're wary of risking side effects in treating a minor problem.

You're also unwilling to succumb to the blandishments of television pitchmen and other media who urge you to take "something" for every ill—a cold, headache, indigestion, constipation, insomnia. These products merely mask symptoms, and there is growing evidence that they interfere with the body's self-healing mechanism.

To escape the risks of synthetic drugs, some people are experimenting with herbs. This route can be dangerous in view of the absence of scientific information about using herbs as medicine. Others are turning to home remedies and discovering that an old tonic owed its curative powers to a generous helping of whiskey.

Faced with these dismal alternatives, it's understandable why persons like yourself are interested in homeopathy and are eager to learn more about it.

Homeopathy is a system of medicine that uses "natural" remedies made from animal, vegetable, and mineral substances. These remedies are prepared in such a way that they are nontoxic and do not cause side effects. (A child could swallow the contents of a bottle and suffer no ill effects.) And the remedies are available at a fraction of the cost of most prescription and nonprescription drugs.

Homeopathic medicine is prescribed according to the law of similars, an age-old principle that recognizes the body's ability to heal itself. This is no newfangled approach to healing; homeopathy was founded in the early 1800s by a German physician and spread rapidly throughout Europe. It was extremely popular in many countries in the nineteenth century, then declined with the use of "wonder drugs" and other changes in the practice of medicine. The holistic movement that surfaced in the early 1970s in America advocates a return to natural laws of healing, and it has sparked a revival of interest in this scientific system of medicine.

This book is written for those of you who do not have a homeopathic physician but want to improve your health and that of your family with homeopathic care. If you have already investigated homeopathy, you know that there are many fine books on the subject —books that describe in depth its principles and practices or offer an account of the author's experiences as a homeopathic physician. Our book is a comprehensive and practical guide to self-help homeopathy. In addition to the homeopathic approach to treating minor ailments and emergencies, we provide proven first-aid procedures and commonsense measures for each condition as well as information about standard drugs and their side effects. Since this book is not intended to replace your physician, throughout the text we point out conditions and emergency situations that are beyond first aid—when to call for medical assistance and what to do while you are awaiting it. And, if you are under the care of a homeopathic physician, we recommend that you do not take any remedies for acute illnesses without checking with your doctor.

Clinical evidence accumulated over more than 150 years of use demonstrates that homeopathic medicine is the viable alternative to standard medicine. You now have access to a scientific system of medicine that is proven safe and effective.

1
What Is Homeopathy?

Homeopathy is a system of medicine whose principles are even older than Hippocrates. It seeks to cure in accordance with natural laws of healing and uses medicines made from natural substances: animal, vegetable, and mineral.

Homeopathy was "discovered" in the early 1800s by a German physician, Samuel Christian Friedrich Hahnemann. Shortly after setting up practice, he became disillusioned with medicine, and with good reason. Eighteenth and nineteenth century physicians believed that sickness was caused by humors, or fluids, that had to be expelled from the body by every possible means. To achieve this end, patients were cauterized, blistered, purged, and bled. Hahnemann protested against these brutal and senseless methods, and his colleagues quickly denounced him for heresy. He was also opposed to the way doctors prescribed medicines. In those days it was customary to mix a great number of drugs in one prescription. In his book, *Who Is Your Doctor and Why?* Dr. Alonzo J. Shadman mentions having seen, in the *Pharmacopoeia* of 1875, a prescription that contained fifty ingredients. Earlier, Hahnemann's outspoken criticism of this "degrading commerce in prescription" naturally enraged the chemists, who were as powerful as our drug companies today, and they were to hound him all of his life.

Hahnemann gave up the practice of medicine and turned to medical translating as a livelihood. But he persisted in his lifelong goal—to discover "if God had not indeed given some law, whereby the diseases of mankind would be cured." His sense of frustration increased when one of his children became critically ill and he could do nothing for her.

It was while translating *Lectures on the Materia Medica* by William Cullen, a Scottish professor of medicine, that Hahnemann stumbled on the key to curing sick people. In this work, the author claimed that cinchona bark, or quinine, cured intermittent fever (malaria) because of its astringent and bitter qualities. This explanation did not sound plausible to Hahnemann, who knew of other substances equally bitter, so he did a daring thing: he tested the medicine on himself.

I took by way of experiment, twice a day, four drachms of good China (quinine). My feet, finger ends, etc. at first became cold; I grew languid and drowsy; then my heart began to palpitate, and my pulse grew hard and small; intolerable anxiety, trembling, prostration throughout all my limbs; then pulsation, in the head, redness of my cheeks, thirst, and, in short, all these symptoms which are ordinarily characteristic of intermittent fever, made their appearance, one after the other, yet without the peculiar chilly, shivering rigor. Briefly, even those symptoms which are of regular occurrence and especially characteristic—as the stupidity of mind, the kind of rigidity in all the limbs, but above all the numb, disagreeable sensation, which seems to have its seat in the periosteum, over every bone in the body—all these make their appearance. This paroxysm lasted two or three hours each time, and recurred if I repeated this dose, not otherwise; I discontinued it, and was in good health.

This was the first "proving", a testing of medicine on a healthy person. The symptoms Hahnemann developed corresponded exactly to the symptoms of malaria. Thus Hahnemann reasoned that malaria was cured by quinine, not because of its bitter taste but owing to the fact that the drug produces the symptoms of malaria in a healthy person.

After experimenting on himself, Hahnemann enlisted the help of friends and followers and embarked on an extensive program of drug testing. When he died at age eighty-eight in 1843, he had conducted or supervised provings on ninety-nine substances. More than 600 other medicines were added to the homeopathic pharmacopoeia by the end of the century.

PRINCIPLES OF HOMEOPATHY

The Law of Similars

The term homeopathy (sometimes spelled homoeopathy) comes from the Greek *homoios* ("similar") and *pathos* ("suffering" or "sickness") The fundamental law upon which homeopathy is based is the *law of similars*, or "Like is cured by like"—in Latin, *similia similibus curentur*. The law of similars states that a remedy can cure a disease if it produces in a healthy person symptoms similar to those of the disease.

Hahnemann did not claim to have discovered the concept. In the tenth century B.C., Hindu sages described the law, as had Hippocrates, who wrote in 400 B.C.: "Through the like, disease is produced and through the application of the like, it is cured." Paracelsus, a sixteenth-century German physician, reiterated the law. Hahnemann, as an erudite thinker, was undoubtedly familiar with these writings, but he was the first to test the principle and establish it as the cornerstone of a system of medicine.

The law works thus in practice: A person develops a fever, with flushed face, dilated pupils, rapid heartbeat, and a feeling of restlessness. The homeopathic physician studies all these symptoms, then searches for a remedy that, under scientifically controlled conditions, has produced all these symptoms in a healthy person. Within a short time after taking the remedy, the fever drops to normal and the person feels well. The law of similars enables the physician to select the one medicine (the *simillimum*) that is needed by matching the symptoms of the individual to the symptoms the remedy induces.

The Law of Proving

The second law of homeopathy, *the law of proving*, refers to the method of testing a substance to determine its medicinal effect. To prove a remedy, each of a group of healthy people is given a dose of the substance daily, and each carefully records the symptoms experienced. Conforming to the standard double-blind method used in pharmacological experiments, approximately half of the test group are used as controls and given an unmedicated tablet or pill (placebo).

When the proving is completed, all the symptoms that the provers consistently experience, such as dizziness, loss of memory, and restlessness, are listed as a characterstic remedy picture in the *Materia Medica,* a prescriber's reference. To treat a patient, the physician looks up the remedy picture in the *Materia Medica,* and, when the symptoms fit, applies the law of similars.

In standard medical practice, drugs are first tested on animals because so many drugs have been found to cause dangerous reactions, even cancer. Homeopaths do not use animals as subjects for testing medicines, since they do not react to chemicals as human beings do. Furthermore, we consider subjective symptoms to be important. And we have no concern about testing homeopathic medicines on healthy human beings because homeopathically prepared remedies are not toxic. The first proving was carried out in 1790, and use of the procedure has continued to the present day. There has never been a report of a lasting adverse drug reaction as the result of a proving.

The Law of Potentization (the Minimum Dose)

The third law of homeopathy, *the law of potentization,* refers to the preparation of a homeopathic remedy. Each is prepared by a controlled process of successive dilutions alternating with succussion (shaking), which may be continued to the point where the resulting medicine contains no molecules of the original substance. These small doses are called *potencies*; lesser dilutions are known as low potencies and greater dilutions as high potencies. As strange as it may seem, the higher the dilution, when prepared in this manner, the greater the potency of the medicine.

In 1800, when the process of potentization was devised, the idea that medicine containing an infinitesimal amount of matter could be curative was inconceivable. In this nuclear age, the power of minute quantities is all too well established. The dose of vitamin B, used to treat certain anemias contains a millionth of a gram of cobalt. Trace elements, present in barely measurable amounts in the body, are essential for its development and functioning. The human body manufactures only fifty to a hundred millionths of a gram of thyroid hormone each day, yet a small excess or deficiency in this already "infinitesimal" amount can seriously affect the health of the individual.

The power of the infinitesimal dose is not clearly understood, but neither is the action of aspirin and many other drugs. The process of potentization makes it possible to use substances such as certain metals, charcoal, and sand, which are inert in their natural state, as medicines. A potentized remedy does not contain sufficient matter to act directly on the tissues, which means that homeopathic medicine is nontoxic and cannot cause side effects. In over 150 years of use, no homeopathic remedy has ever been recalled.

The Single Remedy

Contrary to the current medical practice of frequently prescribing two or more medicines at one time, most homeopaths usually give only one remedy at a time. We are not sure what the effect of two remedies would be, or the interaction between them, but we are sure of the effect of a single remedy. The single remedy has been proved, or tested, on healthy subjects.

The wisdom of the single remedy is pointed up by the ever-increasing problem of drug interactions from multiple prescriptions. In an article in *American Druggist* for September 1978, the author writes: "It has been estimated that during a typical hospital stay, the patient gets an average of ten drugs—and the number sometimes goes as high as thirty or more. Among the ambulatory, nonhospitalized public, it is common for an individual to be taking as many as six different drugs, prescription and nonprescription, at the same time."

The Physician's Desk Reference (PDR) is sprinkled with warnings of potentially dangerous side effects from administration of certain drugs along with others. Taking a random look at my copy of *PDR*, I find a tranquilizer (tranylcypromine sulphate) which carries the warning that use in combination with certain other drugs may result in "hypertension headache and related symptoms... hypertensive crises or severe convulsive seizures." Such sedative-hypnotics are the most prescribed medications in the world.

Safe, but Why Effective?

Numerous theories have been offered as to why homeopathic remedies work. A 1954 newspaper report describing the research of the late Dr. William E. Boyd of Glasgow contained this explanation: "The power of the solution does not depend solely on the degree of dilution but on a special progressive method in its preparation; the energy latent in the drug is apparently liberated and increased by a forceful shaking of the liquid at each stage of the process."

Dr. F.K. Bellokossy of Denver compares the process of potentizing a homeopathic drug—shaking a dilution or grinding powdered dry materials—to magnetizing a glass rod by rubbing it. "We thus produce electric fields around every particle of the powdered drug; and the more we triturate (grind), the stronger electric fields we produce, and the more potentized becomes the triturated material."

At present, there is no widely accepted theory to explain why homeopathic medicine works, but with physicists taking an active interest in homeopathy, such an explanation seems imminent. One of these physicists is Dr. William A. Tiller, professor in the Department of Materials Science and Engineering, Stanford University. In a letter to one of the authors, he writes:

> As humankind evolves, the individual becomes a more integrated and finely tuned system and more sensitive with respect to changes in subtle energies. Our future medicine will proceed towards the development of techniques and treatments that use successively finer and finer energies... In my modeling, homeopathic remedies treat at the etheric level of substance. ("Etheric" means not directly observable via our physical senses or instruments.) Since this method of treatment is already in use and is easy to practice, I expect it to flourish in the near future while allopathic (standard) medicine declines.

A COMPARISON OF HOMEOPATHY AND STANDARD MEDICINE (ALLOPATHY)

Meaning of Symptoms

The homeopath believes that the body is always striving to keep itself healthy, or in balance, just as a keel coat attempts to right itself in the water. The force that acts in this protective manner is called the vital force. When the body is threatened by harmful external forces, the vital force, or defense mechanism, produces symptoms such as pain, fever, mucus, cough. These symptoms, although unpleasant for the patient, have a purpose: to restore harmony or balance. Pain is a warning that something is wrong. Fever inactivates many viruses that attack the body. Mucus is produced in the respiratory tract to surround and carry off irritating material. A cough expels the mucus that would otherwise hinder breathing.

A homeopathic physician regards symptoms as a healthy reaction of the body's defense mechanism to harmful forces; such symptoms need to be supported rather than interfered with. Standard medicine takes a different view; it regards symptoms as manifestations of the disease, to be opposed or suppressed. Aspirin or other antifever drugs are given to lower fever, antihistamine to dry up nasal secretions, cough syrup to suppress a cough.

Meaning of Disease

Because symptoms that reflect the body's condition are constantly changing, homeopaths regard disease, or disharmony of the body, as a dynamic condition. We treat the patient according to the symptoms, not according to the "disease." This is contrary to the standard view of disease as an entity unto itself. The allopathic doctor elicits the patient's symptoms and attempts to group them under a known diagnosis. He or she then prescribes the treatment established for that disease.

The Body, Not the Germs

We're always surrounded by germs, inside our body, in our food, in the air we breathe. In the battle raging between the body and invading forces, the homeopath is not primarily concerned with identifying the enemy—the type of bacteria. Our aim is to strengthen the body so it can resist these harmful organisms. In standard medicine, on the other hand, the goal is to identify the invader and select a powerful drug to destroy the specific germ.

Holistic Approach versus Specialization

We believe that all parts of the body are interdependent, and therefore we treat the patient as a whole person, rather than concentrating on one organ or one part of the body. We do not attempt to separate mental from physical illness; all are symptoms of the individual. Homeopathy is truly holistic, and has been since its inception 180 years ago.

For centuries, standard medicine has taken a different approach; it treats a patient's mind and body as separate entities. A speaker at a holistic health conference recently quipped that in modern medicine the general practitioner treats the body, sends the head to a shrink and the soul to a clergyman.

Attitude of the Physician

The concept of the vital force, an age-old belief in the body's guiding intelligence, instills an attitude of humility in the homeopathic physician. We accept the fact that we cannot comprehend all the marvelous and complex workings of the body and aim to assist it as best we can. In the nineteenth century, when homeopathy was founded, the conventional physician believed his wisdom was greater than that of the body, and subjected the patient to extreme and often fatal measures, such as bloodletting. The current practice of giving the patient powerful drugs that often produce harmful side effects and cause other diseases represents a continuation of this attitude.

No one would mistake homeopathy for allopathy, but sometimes people confuse homeopathy with naturopathy or herbalism because of their apparent similarities.

HOMEOPATHY AND NATUROPATHY

Both the naturopath and the homeopath believe in the healing power of Nature, Hippocrates' *Vis Medicatrix Naturae*, or vital force. The naturopath emphasizes the importance of diet, fresh air, exercise, and peace of mind, as does the homeopath. Naturopathy is also holistic; the naturopath treats the whole person in an effort to find the cause of illness, rather than merely removing symptoms.

Preventive medicine and a holistic approach are important, but homeopathy alone is a science that operates systematically. As Harris L. Coulter says in his introduction to *Homeopathic Medicine*, the laws of homeopathy "enable the physician to understand the patient's illness and to prescribe the drug that will act curatively." The crucial difference between the two systems is that homeopathy, as Coulter defines it, is a "system of drug therapy, a set of rules governing the administration of drugs to sick people."

Naturopaths are licensed to practice in several states. However homeopaths are medical doctors and as such are licensed to practice in all states.

HOMEOPATHY AND HERBALISM

People sometimes confuse homeopathy and herbalism because both systems use herbs as medicines. Their methods of preparing these materials, however, are very different. The herbalist may use an age-old formula for making an herb tea or a poultice, but can also improvise in the manner of an experienced cook departing from a recipe. As one herbalist expressed it, "Herbalism is more an art and a tool of divine nature than a science . . . . It is very difficult for an herbalist to tell specifically why he would use this or that herb in a formula." In this system that depends on the herbalist's intuition and experience, it is standard practice to increase the effect of a formula by combining a number of herbs.

This "artistic" approach to preparing medicine has its dangers. A great many medicinal herbs are toxic, particularly when the person ingests a large amount. But the self-help herbalist has no way of knowing what constitutes a "safe" dose, since this information is seldom provided in herb books. In the *Journal of the American Medical Association*, a doctor recently reported three cases of poisoning, one fatal, resulting from three young women, independently, dosing themselves with large amounts of oil from the pennyroyal plant.

Homeopathy bears no relation to the free-spirit approach and practices of herbalism. Homeopathy is scientific medicine; its rule were developed by following the procedures of the scientific method. Homeopathic medications are prepared according to an exact process and prescribed according to the law of similars. A physician usually administers only a single remedy at one time. Finally, although many homeopathic remedies are made from poisonous herbs or plants, the potentized remedy contains only minute amounts of the original substance and is nontoxic.

HOMEOPATHY SUPPRESSED IN AMERICA

If homeopathy is such an advanced system of medicine, why is it not more widely practiced?

Many people today do not realize that in America homeopathy was widely practiced in the latter half of the nineteenth century. In 1890, there were 14,000 homeopaths as compared to 100,000 conventional physicians. In some areas—New England, the Middle Atlantic States, and the Midwest—one out of four or five physicians was a homeopath. There were twenty-two homeopathic medical schools and over a hundred homeopathic hospitals. The elite of every community—the social, intellectual, political, and business leaders—patronized the homeopaths.

Homeopathy was first introduced in America as a result of its success in treating the cholera epidemic of 1832 in Europe. Our country was ripe for a new and humane system of medicine. The regular physician had two standard methods of treatment. One was to administer huge, or "heroic," doses of mercurous chloride, known as "calomel," to purge patients. This frequently caused the patient continuous salivation accompanied by swelling of the tongue. Patients also frequently lost all their teeth and, in extreme cases of mercurial poisoning, were unable to open their mouths. The other treatment that the physician used for every disease was bloodletting. The eminent Dr. Benjamin Rush (for whom a hospital in Philadelphia was named, as well as the Rush Medical College in Chicago) advised: "Bleeding should be continued . . until four fifths of the blood contained in the body are drawn away." Children including newborns, were also bled routinely.

So it is understandable why the homeopaths immediately attracted patients. In place of these barbaric methods, they had dozens of different remedies, none of which caused any disagreeable side effects. As proof that the homeopath's sweet-tasting white granules, often called "little sugar pills," were effective, a large number of homeopathic remedies were adopted by the allopaths, and some are still being used today. One of the best known is nitroglycerine, used in certain heart ailments.

The medical establishment was hostile to homeopathy from the time it was introduced into the United States. In the 1830s and 40s, when the public was dissatisfied with the harsh practices of regular medicine, homeopathy was not the only "alternative thereapy"; botanical medicine and Thomsonian naturopathy were also popular. But homeopathy posed the greatest threat to orthodox medicine because its practitioners were licensed medical doctors. It was galling to the establishment that these homeopathic physicians, well trained in orthodox medicine, were critical of the system and had "defected" to homeopathy.

The establishment promptly took strong measures to suppress this upstart discipline.

The American Medical Association (AMA) was formed in 1846 as a direct response to the American Institute of Homeopathy two years earlier. Homeopaths were denied admittance to standard medical societies. A member of such a society who consulted with a homeopath was punished by ostracism and expulsion. (In 1878, a physician was expelled from a medical society in Connecticut for consulting with a homeopath—his wife!) The hostility increased as "the best people" flocked to the homeopaths, and the regular physicians felt the pinch in their pocketbooks.

What killed, or almost killed, homeopathy? One reason for its decline was the changing life-style in America. The homeopathic physician was the quintessence of the family doctor who knew patients and their families intimately and could afford to devote a good deal of time to them, since most would remain patients for life. The shift to a mobile urban society as well as the rise of specialization changed that pattern. Homeopathic prescribing, which demands both time and intellectual effort, became increasingly out of step with the tempo of the times.

The rise of the drug industry after the Civil War further changed the practice of medicine. The allopath could now buy a proprietary, or compound, drug that saved time and effort, while the homeopath, opposed to any mixing of medicines, continued prescribing medicines in the same "old-fashioned" way. As medical historian Harris L. Coulter points out, "The pharmaceutical industry . . . in the 1890s and early 1900s allied with the American Medical Association in its [the medical association's] final campaign against homeopathy."

A further severe blow to homeopathy was the Flexner Report in 1910, an evaluation of medical schools by the AMA. In view of the AMA's traditional opposition to "sectarian medicine," it is not surprising that the examiners gave a low rating to homeopathic medical schools, among others, thus denying them a share in the millions of dollars, principally the Rockefeller grants, that were being given to allopathic institutions. One by one, the homeopathic medical schools closed and the homeopathic hospitals were converted to standard institutions. Flower Fifth Avenue Hospital and Medical College became New York Medical College; Hahnemann Hospital in San Francisco was recently renamed the Marshall Hale Hospital. With the advent of the "wonder drugs" in the early 1940s, homeopathy appeared to be obsolete.

HOMEOPATHY : THE ALTERNATIVE OF THE FUTURE

This dismal prospect is rapidly changing. In an article written in 1970, Harris L. Coulter points out that we are witnessing a popular revolt against orthodox medical practices "comparable to the revolt of the 1830s and 1840s which ensconced homeopathy on the American medical scene."

This revolt has gathered steam with the emergence of holistic health, a movement that surfaced in California in the early 1970s. Its practitioners, trained in a variety of disciplines, hold the common belief that medicine has become divorced from natural healing. According to Edward Bauman, coeditor of *The Holistic Health Handbook*, "Holistic health is a sympathetic response to the distrust and frustration engendered by specialized allopathic medicine." Holistic therapists criticize widespread use of dangerous drugs, the dehumanizing effect of specialization, the failure to cure chronic degenerative disease. The conventional physician prescribes drugs to alleviate the symptoms of arthritis, diabetes, emphysema, but this treatment fails to attack the root of the problem.

Holistic-minded professionals were amazed to stumble upon homeopathy. Here was a "natural" system of medicine that used no toxic drugs, treated the whole person, and, in many instances, cured "hopeless" chronic conditions. Furthermore, the efficacy of homeopathy had been demonstrated by the clinical experience of physicians for over 150 years.

So, with health a national preoccupation, homeopathy is emerging as a vigorous alternative to standard medicine. An increasing number of physicians and nurses are enrolling in the summer course offered by the National Center for Homeopathy. People are investigating homeopathy and incorporating it into their lives. Lay people all over the country are forming homeopathic study groups.

Homeopathy is alive and well in other parts of the world. In Britain, members of the Royal Family have been cared for by homeopathic physicians since the reign of Queen Victoria. There are around 200 homeopathic physicians in Britain; the principal hospitals offering such treatment are in London and Glasgow. France has nearly 800 homeopathic physicians, and the movement is also active in Germany, Austria, and Switzerland.

India is a stronghold of homeopathy, with 124 homeopathic medical schools. Central and Latin America are also important centers. In Mexico there are three homeopathic medical colleges, two of which are state supported. There is a similar school of medicine in Brazil, and the medical school in Santiago, Chile, includes a professor of homeopathy. Around 450 Argentine physicians are homeopaths.

Homeopathy is on the rise all over the world, owing to the dissatisfaction of both physician and patient with the medical treatment at their disposal. Both are looking for a safe and effective approach to healing and finding the answer in homeopathy.

In the next chapter you'll learn how one homeopath practices medicine and what it's like to be a homeopathic patient.

2
A Homeopathic Physician at Work

THE other day, a new patient, a wiry older lady, said to me, "I don't like going to doctors. You're not a medical doctor, are you?" I had to admit I was a "real" doctor and pointed to my diploma from the College of Medicine of the Ohio State University.

Many are uncertain about a homeopath's training. A homeopathic physician in America undergoes the same training as any other doctor of medicine; he or she is a graduate of an accredited medical college, receives an M.D. degree, and is licensed by the state. To learn the specialty of homeopathy, sometimes called homeotherapeutics, the doctor takes a postgraduate course in the subject, then a preceptorship with a practicing homeopathic physician.

TAKING THE CASE

Although each homeopathic physician has his or her own way of practicing, homeopathy is a system of medicine with clearly defined principles and methodology, and there is an element of standardization. "Taking the case," which means eliciting all the necessary information about a patient, adheres to a form as exacting as a Japanese tea ceremony.

To understand how I practice medicine, imagine you are seated in my waiting room. My office is in a wing of my home. On an average day, there's pleasant air of sociability in the waiting room. A farmer chats with a banker from town; a grandmotherly lady talks playfully with an infant held in his mother's arms.

Close to the hour, I come down the steps to fetch my next patient, Mr. Smith. He is a new patient, and I know from our telephone conversation that he is in his early 40s and has stomach trouble. Why don't I send my secretary, Anne? I don't like to have a patient ushered into my office—it creates the impression of the doctor as an authority figure—but, more important, this first glimpse of a patient tells me a good deal about him. Mr. Smith, well dressed, with a sallow complexion, sits frowning, hands slightly clenched. It takes no student of body language to see that he is tense and anxious.

He follows me up the steep stairs to my small, book-cluttered consulting room. I begin by filling out the patient form—age, marital status, date and place of birth. Again, why don't I have my secretary do this? My aim in this interview is to learn everything I can about this patient in order to select the remedy that will match all his symptoms. These routine questions serve as a springboard. Mr. Smith was born in Dayton. I ask, Did you go to school here? Yes, he went to a local high school and, yes, he was a good student. "I had to be," he smiles wryly, "my parents wouldn't stand for anything less than A's." Already I know something about him—exacting, ambitious parents. The pattern of driving himself to succeed began at an early age.

The form completed, I ask, What is troubling you? "My stomach," he says. How does it trouble you? "About a half hour after dinner, it hurts and I feel sick as if I'm going to vomit." What else? "I get a lot of headaches." What's your headache like? "A dull pressure in my forehead." Anything else? He reveals that he is constipated—"I have the urge but can't go"—troubled with gas, belching, a bitter taste in his mouth. I let the patient talk freely, interjecting only an occasional "What else?" until he has described all his problems.

Then I go back over each symptom. When did his stomach problem first occur? What time of day is it better or worse? How does weather affect his indigestion; does he like being in a warm room or is he more comfortable out-of-doors? Does he feel better or worse in cold, damp weather? Is the pain worse on the left or right side?

The patient's food preferences are important. He tells me he likes Mexican food. I note, "Likes highly spiced food." He loves coffee, although it doesn't agree with him. He's in the habit of drinking several cocktails at lunch and dinner, even though liquor brings on a headache and indigestion. He used to like beer but now can't stand the taste. How about thirst? Does he often get up from his desk to drink water?

I ask him about his forebears. What illnesses run in his family? Did some of his ancestors live to a ripe old age? The answers to these questions will indicate his inheritance of vitality and strength.

Now that we are comfortable with each other, I ask about his emotional state, his mental symptoms. He tells me that he is extremely irritable, can't tolerate criticism, can't stand noise. His concentration has fallen off, he worries a lot. Little by little the pieces fit together to form a portrait. By the end of our hour-long session, I have a clear picture of this man—not only his stomachache or his headache, but Mr. Smith as an individual.

Seated in the consultation room after his physical examination, Mr. Smith asks, "Do I have an ulcer?" No, I tell him, but you've had more stress than your body can handle and this has affected your whole system, throwing it out of balance. If Mr. Smith needs a diagnosis for insurance purposes, I can produce one: dyspepsia. But I don't need a diagnosis to help this patient. I am going to treat Mr. Smith according to his individual symptoms, produced by his defense mechanism, which reflect the changes taking place in his system. By doing so, I can hope to reverse the trend of his disease before it causes pathological changes.

Needing time to reflect on Mr. Smith's case, I ask him to return the following week.

Later, looking over my voluminous notes concerning Mr. Smith, I note the strong symptoms that I've underlined. These are the ones that really bother him, such as "pain after eating" and "nausea after eating." I have also underlined his those unusual symptoms, we call "strange, rare, and peculiar," that reflect his individual response to what is troubling him. One of these is "aversion to beer."

Out of a dozen "strong" symptoms, five stand out. Because there are approximately

500 remedies in daily use, each with a multitude of symptoms, it is impossible to carry all this information in one's head. There is an index to the symptoms and their remedies known as the *Repertory of the Homeopathic Materia Medica* by James Tyler Kent, M.D. This book is the daily companion of most the world's practicing homeopathic physicians, and I turn to it now to look up Mr. Smith's strong symptoms.

"Nausea after eating" shows four remedies, one of which is *Nux vomica*, made from the seeds of the poison nut. The second symptom, "pain after eating," shows the same four remedies and several others. The third symptom, "dull headache in the morning," lists *Nux* as one of its remedies. The remaining two strong symptoms, "worse from drinking coffee" and "ineffectual urging to move the bowels," also list *Nux* as one of the remedies.

Nux vomica having been indicated for each of these five symptoms, I turn to the *Materia Medica*, the book that describes each remedy in detail, and read the description of *Nux*. The *Materia Medica* is a description of the symptoms that each medicine has produced in healthy people. These symptoms are expressed in the provers' own words rather than in the medical jargon of the time. That is why it is important for me to encourage my patients to speak freely about their feelings. Over the past 150 years, there have been minor changes in speech patterns, but people still hurt in the same way.

According to the *Materia Medica*, the *Nux vomica* patient is "thin, spare, quick, active, nervous, and irritable. . ." Here is a perfect description of my patient. The *Repertory* led me to the right remedy and the *Materia Medica* confirms the selection.

On Mr. Smith's return visit, I give him a single high potency dose of *Nux vomica* and ask that he report any changes. I recommend that he eliminate coffee, which may interfere with the action of the remedy.

Two days later, Mr. Smith's wife calls. Her husband came home from work last evening complaining of a terrible stomachache. No, he didn't seem as irritable, she said. He even jocked that the medicine had made him sicker. I reassure her that his temporary upset is a normal response.

On his next visit, two weeks later, Mr. Smith tells me that the medicine "shook him up" but he's feeling fine now. "I haven't had any stomach pains or headache and I'm less irritable."

Mr. Smith's response illustrates the classic homeopathic "aggravation," a sign that the remedy is stimulating the patient's defense mechanism. The sick person is always ultrasensitive to his similar remedy. Just as a tuning fork responds by resonating to the properly struck note, so the individual given the similar medicine responds with an increase of all symptoms. **I am always happy to have a patient report an aggravation, as this usually shows that the remedy was the right one. An aggravation generally lasts a day or two and is followed by improvement.**

During this last visit, I talk with Mr. Smith about the importance of changing his lifestyle—cutting down his alcohol intake, exercising more, learning to recognize tension and deal with it. The remedy, I explain, can help bring your system into balance, but if you continue to abuse your body, you'll be in trouble again.

Not every person with an upset stomach, aching head, and irritability will benefit from *Nux vomica*; I chose *Nux* for Mr. Smith because the symptoms produced by this remedy matched all of his symptoms. *Nux*, being the most similar remedy, or the *simillimum*, will stimulate Mr. Smith's defense mechanism that is producing these symptoms in an effort to restore harmony. Once his system is in balance, the symptoms will subside because they are no longer needed.

The foregoing is an example of "constitutional prescribing," i.e., prescribing for **a chronic ailment—one that will not get better by itself. It is not directed at the disease or even at the patient's chief complaint, but at the whole being of the person.** The correct constitutional remedy acts instantaneously, like an electric spark, upon the defense mechanism or vital force; the effects of one dose may last for months. Therefore, when a person is under constitutional treatment, he or she must not take any other homeopathic medicine without consulting the doctor. Taking another remedy while under the influence of a contitutional prescription may so confuse the patient's symptoms that it becomes almost impossible to untangle the case.

THE MAKING OF A HOMEOPATH

I had the good fortune to be born into a homeopathic family. My father, Dr. Edmund Prior Banning, was a homeopathic physician, and, unbelievable as it sounds, fought in the Civil War. He was sixty-five when I was born and acquired a protégé, John Panos, when I was a little girl. John was a young Greek immigrant who yearned to be a doctor and with my father's help, managed to achieve his goal. After many years, John and I were married. We had two daughters, but our happy life together was short. John's years of incessant work and study took their toll, and he died of a heart attack at age forty-seven.

John's patients, like lost sheep, sought my advice on their medical problems. Despite my lifetime exposure to homeopathy, I knew very little about the science and could do nothing to help them. Determined to rectify this, I enrolled in a premedical program at the University of Dayton and then attended Ohio State University College of Medicine. After graduating from medical school and completing internship and residency, I assisted Dr. Julia Green, a renownd homeopath, then eighty years old, in Washington, D.C. Later, I opened my own office in that city, and after that, in Tipp City, Ohio.

HOMEOPATHY VERSUS ALLOPATHY: A PRACTICAL VIEW

Now that you've seen me at work, you have a better idea of how a homeopathic physician differs from a standard general practitioner. Chapter 1 listed some of the theoretical differences between homeopathy and allopathy. It's now time for a closer look.

A homeopath spends more time with each patient and sees fewer patients. I spend at least an hour with a new patient. To prescribe for my patient on the basis of all symptoms, I must know that person as an individual—his or her emotional and mental symptoms as well as the physical ones. Consequently, I limit myself to about ten patients per day. One general practitioner tells me he spends about ten minutes with each patient and sees thirty to forty patients per day.

Homeopathic treatment is less expensive, involving fewer doctor visits. My hourly fee is, I believe, comparable to that of any other general practitioner; but my patients who were formerly cared for by a conventional family practitioner tell me they have fewer office visits because they do not get sick as often. The most encouraging evidence of the value of homeopathic treatment is shown by patients in whose families homeopathy has been a tradition for several generations. Elsie, age seventy-five and a fourth-generation homeopathic patient, amazes all her friends with her energy and vitality. In those rare instances when she contracts an acute disease, she throws it off very quickly.

Homeopathic treatment involves fewer diagnostic studies. According to the Department of Health and Human Services, each doctor generates $ 200,000 in patient medical costs a year. This does not include charges for physicians' services but consists of bills paid for drugs, surgery, hospitalization, and other medical procedures. The homeopath is less apt to subject a patient to such expenses.

I use x-ray and laboratory tests, but to a much lesser extent than the conventional physician. This is according to our belief that the disease process first affects the vital force, or defense mechanism, and this alteration manifests itself as symptoms that precede any measurable changes in the person's blood or tissues. (Often a person seeking help from an ordinary doctor will say, "I don't feel right but the doctor can't find anything wrong.") Treating on the basis of the totality of symptoms gives us a chance to reverse the disease process *before* any pathological changes occur.

The traditional physician is interested in symptoms but relies more on objective evidence. He does not make a diagnosis of anemia, for example, before he sees the results of the blood test. If we are treating a person whose symptoms point to anemia, we like to have a blood test confirm this diagnosis. But we don't need this objective evidence in order to treat the patient, because we are not treating anemia but rather the patient as a whole.

Homeopathic medicine is inexpensive. Homeopathic medicines are normally quite cheap. One reason for the low cost of medicine is that homeopathic pharmaceutical companies have few research expenses: *All* of the remedies, around 500 in common use, have been proven and reproven over the past 150 years. Another factor keeping the cost low is the absence of promotional expenses. The pharmacies that manufacture and dispense homeopathic medicine, are low-key operations that have no need to spend vast sums in alerting prescribing doctors to new drugs. Except for some minor additions, the current *Homeopathic Pharmacopoeia of the U.S.* contains the same medicines as the first edition in 1832.

Allopathic drugs, on the other hand, cost a good deal more than homeopathic medicine. New drugs are particularly expensive because of the investment they demand in research and development. According to a representative of the Pharmaceutical Manufacturers Association, the expense of launching a new drug is about $ 55 million. The majority of them, however, to quote Milton Silverman and Philip Lee, authors of *Pills, Profits and Politics*, are "me-too" items—minor modifications of existing products that are merely new, not necessarily better.

Obviously, as Walter Modell, Professor of Pharmacology at the Cornell University Medical College, points out in his book, *Drugs*, keeping track of all these new drugs is far beyond the capacity of a practicing physician. My allopathic colleague has available for prescription a total of about 10,000 drugs. I select from about 500 remedies, most of which I know more or less intimately.

A homeopathic remedy does not cause side effects. When I prescribe a remedy, I don't have to worry, Is this drug safe? I have never heard of a homeopathic medicine being recalled for causing adverse side effects, which is an enviable record considering that these remedies have been in use for more than 150 years.

My allopathic colleagues have no such assurance of safety. Adverse drug reactions rank among the top ten causes of hospitalization. As many as 28 percent of the 30 million patients hospitalized annually in America may suffer an adverse reaction. Serious drug reactions are estimated at from 5 million to 10 million a year.

These statistics only bear out what we have been reading in newspapers and magazines. To quote some recent stories: "Cancer researchers say reserpine, a widely used high blood pressure drug, has caused cancer in rats. . . . Methapyrilene, an antihistamine used in over-the-counter sleeping preparations, has been banned by the Food and Drug Administration as a carcinogen. . . . Tagamet, an ulcer remedy introduced in 1976 and one of the most widely used prescription drugs, may have cancer-causing side effects. . . . Antiarrhythmic agents (for an irregular heartbeat) may cause sudden death. . . . New evidence suggests that Valium, the U.S.'s most widely prescribed pill (50 million prescriptions a year), may be addictive even if taken only briefly. . . ."

THE SATISFACTION OF HOMEOPATHY

I have never regretted choosing homeopathy as a specialty, even though the medical establishment persists in regarding us as "fringe" practitioners. I had a taste of this shortly after I opened my office near Tipp City in 1972. I needed an internist to care for an ill patient while I attended an out-of-town medical meeting and called a physician who had been highly recommended by a colleague. The internist readily agreed to see my patient, apologized profusely for not having called me when I first moved to the area, and invited me to the next county medical society meeting.

Shortly after I returned, I received a report from the internist about my patient, but no personal message or mention of the forthcoming meeting. Could my patient have talked excessively about the virtues of homeopathic treatment? Did the internist feel uncomfortable about associating with a homeopathic physician? I'll never know.

But the advantages of being a homeopath far outweigh the disadvantages. It is such a satisfaction to treat patients with safe and effective remedies. A succession of patients come to mind, such as twelve-year-old Roger whom I treated for the first time this past winter. He had flu symptoms—a dry, painful cough, sore chest, bursting headache—that had lingered for some time. The physician who had been treating him had prescribed aspirin and cough syrup, which only relieved the symptoms temporarily. I prescribed a remedy that matched all of Roger's symptoms, and within a day or two he was well.

The greatest satisfaction comes from treating patients with chronic conditions. James, a husky fifty-year-old farmer, complained of puffy, stiff hands; it was increasingly difficult for him to make a fist and grasp things. I prescribed *Rhus toxicodendron*, a remedy that is often indicated for arthritis. On his next visit, James showed me that he had more strength in his hand and felt better in general.

Doris, a patient, recently brought her mother, Mrs. W., to see me. As Doris had explained on the phone, her mother suffered from sciatica—pain in the sacroiliac and running down the back of her leg to her foot. "I hope you can help her," Doris said with a sigh.

Despite her pain, Mrs. W. seemed extremely pleasant and cheerful during our interview. I felt sure that she needed *Colocynth*—all her symptoms pointed to this remedy, except that Mrs. W. didn't exhibit the disagreeable personality that is characteristic of this remedy. I excused myself and went down to the waiting room. I asked Doris, Does your mother have a good disposition? The answer was a thundering "No!" I prescribed high potency *Colocynth*

(Bitter Apple), and within a few days, Mrs. W.'s pain had lessened. A month later, when Mrs. W. came in for a follow up visit, she was almost free of pain, and according to her daughter, her disposition had improved as well.

Of course, we don't always succeed, at least on the first attempt. Now and then, I prescribe the "wrong" remedy, one that does not match all of the patient's symptoms, and the result is that nothing happens. *Contrary to the case with allopathic drugs, the wrong homeopathic remedy will do no harm*; at worst, I have wasted the patient's time. These occasional failures do not shake my faith in homeopathy but spur me to try harder next time. As Constantine Hering, a great nineteenth-century homeopath, said, "It is not the medicine that fails, but the physician who prescribes it."

One of the pleasures of being a homeopathic physician is the close relationship with my patients that makes it easier for me to help them. When Mrs. S. calls me about "that shooting pain in my neck," I can usually predict that she is anticipating a visit from her mother-in-law. Mrs. S., in turn, knows that at the end of August I am apt to be depleted after teaching a postgraduate course and makes allowances for my less than alert behaviour.

This mutual understanding and affection are not so prevalent in conventional medicine. According to reports in the press and elsewhere, the public feels **that medical care has become impersonal, too costly; and there is growing mistrust of prescription drugs and their potential side effects.** Evidence of this attitude is the rise in medical malpractice suits, which are increasing at a rate of about 10 percent a year in the United States.

Why the difference in the two systems? A close doctor-patient relationship is essential to homeopathy. We treat the patient, not the disease, which means getting to know every patient as an individual—knowing that person's feelings, thoughts, and family situation. You can describe this approach as either "holistic" or a return to the old-fashioned family doctor.

The active role that the homeopathic patient plays in the healing process also contributes to an egalitarian relationship of the best kind. The patient must report symptoms accurately in order to guide the physician to the correct remedy. This entails phone calls, discussions—a far cry from the passive "heal me" patient role.

The type of person who is attracted to homeopathy favors a close, harmonious relationship. In a study based on a small sample of homeopathic patients, Robert A. Alvina and Laurence J. Schneiderman sketched a profile of the average patient, whose thinking goes like this: "I want to avoid taking traditional drugs. I realize that health is not a matter of popping pills but involves diet, exercise, and positive thinking. I want to take responsibility for my own health and visualize my doctor as a resource person who can help me." This is the mature individual whom I seem to attract and enjoy treating.

As you may have already surmised, practicing homeopathy is both a science and an art that demand a lifetime of study. But self-help homeopathy—the subject of this book—is one that any person concerned with better health can master. It requires learning the principles of homeopathy, described in chapter 1, and familiarizing yourself with the remedies most frequently indicated for minor ailments and emergencies. In most cases, it is a simple matter to limit the degree of discomfort and prevent future trouble.

In the next chapter, you will learn about the twenty-eight homeopathic remedies in the Home Remedy Kit and how to use them.

3

Your Home Remedy Kit

IF you believe in the motto "Be prepared," you undoubtedly have a box containing first-aid equipment—bandages, gauze pads, alcohol, a thermometer—in your bathroom. In addition, if you're new to homeopathy, your medical supplies probably include an antibiotic ointment, merthiolate, syrup of *Ipecac*, and an eyewash.

The homeopathic Home Remedy Kit, containing twenty-eight of the most frequently indicated remedies, is quite different from the usual medicine chest. Although some items in the Home Remedy Kit have specific uses in emergency situations, the scope of the kit goes beyond first-aid measures. I can best explain this by telling you how the kit came about.

When I was practicing in Washington, D.C., some of my patients, many of whom lived several hours' drive from my office, asked me to give a study course in homeopathy. They wanted a better understanding of the subject and, in the event of an acute illness or emergency, needed to have their remedies on hand and to know how to prescribe them. I subsequently gave such a course and helped each member assemble a kit.

At first, when confronted with the need for homeopathic treatment, each kit holder conferred with me by telephone. But as each gained experience, the calls became less frequent. Some time afterwards, I moved to Ohio. A year later, when I returned to Washington for a visit and had a reunion with my "students," I was delighted to find that each had dealt very competently with her respective acute medical problems. This experience stimulated our making the Home Remedy Kit available to the public. Accompanying the kit is a lecture series in pamphlet form based on the original study course I gave in Washington, D.C.

Medical self-help is part of the American tradition. There were few doctors in the colonial period, and in those days the public was extremely skeptical of doctors, with good reason. Like their European counterparts, the American physician's standard form of treatment was to bleed a patient. Consequently, most colonial families relied on a home remedy kit of botanical medicines. In the fall, the mistress of the house gathered herbs such as horehound, sassafras and dandelion, which she dried and hung for future use. When someone became ill, she used these herbs to concoct a remedy to meet the need.

Nearly every community had its "goodwife" who supplemented her storehouse of English herbal medicines, plasters, and ointments with medicinal herbs acquired from her

Indian neighbours. She decocted (prepared by boiling) the wintergreen plant and prescribed the infusion as a diuretic (to increase excretion of urine). Yaupon holly was used to stimulate the heart, and the Indians' balsam root for coughs and colds. In some regions the favored remedy for diarrhea and dysentery was "Indian chocolate," made by decocting the root of an herb called water avens and adding honey and milk to the decoction.

As civilization moved westward, the pioneer woman prescribed for her household and often doctored other families. Old diaries and letters testify to the skill and courage of these women who, equipped with a home doctoring book and home remedies, rode great distances on horseback to treat sick neighbors and deliver babies.

A popular "doctor book" in nineteenth-century America was *A Guide to Homeopathic Practice Designed for the Use of Families and Private Individuals* by I. D. Johnson, M.D. Another was Dr. Constantine Hering's *Domestic Physician*, a two-volume materia medica, first published in 1835. Families who wanted to treat themselves homeopathically could obtain a "domestic kit," a set of around forty homeopathic remedies, along with the *Domestic Physician*, for five dollars.

According to medical historian Harris L. Coulter, "These domestic kits were the mainstay of the female practitioner, and their influence on the spread of homeopathy was gigantic." The kit gained popularity through the decades, and by the 1870s and 1880 was a fixture in thousands of households.

A growing number of Americans want to continue this tradition of assuming greater responsibility for their health. Grace and Bill, a wife and husband who live on a farm in Arkansas, exemplify this spirit. Some years ago, as graduate students in Ohio searching for a lifestyle as free as possible of pollution, this couple discovered homeopathy and knew it was right for them. They read widely on the subject and, at some point, chose me as their family doctor. Shortly before moving to Arkansas, they came in for a checkup as their pioneer forebears might have done before the westward journey. I prescribed a constitutional remedy for each and helped them select remedies for their extensive home remedy kit.

With the help of homeopathic remedies, Bill and Grace, now the parents of two young daughters, cope with everyday ailments and emergencies. Poison ivy in that area is a real problem, Bill says. He used to suffer badly from it until he learned about *Rhus toxicodendron*, a remedy made from the poison ivy plant. "*Rhus tox* clears it right up," Bill said.

Building their own house led to a multitude of accidents. "One day, a 300 pound scaffold fell on my ankle. The whole side of my leg turned purple." Bill took *Arnica* internally and Grace regularly applied *Arnica* tincture to the injured leg. "The leg didn't swell up and two days later I was walking," Bill said.

Their home remedy kit doesn't replace my services. Bill or Grace calls me promptly when they suspect that a medical problem is serious. But having their remedies close at hand and knowing when and how to use them is a constant comfort and, in many instances, probably averts a more serious illness.

THE HOMEOPATHIC HOUSEHOLD KIT

The Homeopathic Home Remedy Kit contains twenty-eight remedies—those most frequently indicated for treating minor ailments and injuries. This is by no means a complete list; as time goes by you may wish to add others. I have a black bag stocked with 144 remedies, and yet I often need one that is not in my bag. For the present, however, we believe this group of carefully selected remedies will make a good start toward meeting your everyday needs.

Homeopathic remedies are supplied in various forms—tablets, granules, and tinctures. Most people prefer the tablet form, in which an alcoholic solution, or dilution, is poured into specially prepared sugar granules that absorb the medication as the alcohol evaporates. Granules are in powder form and are the safest way to administer a remedy if the patient is unconscious. A tincture is an alcoholic solution. Since the concentration of alcohol in a tincture can be irritating, we use the tincture to prepare a lotion as an external remedy to wash and heal the skin. (Another reason for using lotion rather than tincture is to conserve one's supply of tincture.)

The twenty-eight remedies in the kit are in tablet form; each vial, clearly labeled, contains 125 tablets. Vials are stored in a $3\frac{1}{2} \times 6$-inch plastic box with a snap lock. Accompanying the kit are six pamphlets, *Family Self-Help Using Homeopathy* (the Washington study course), and a booklet that briefly describes the use of homeopathic medicine.

Inside Your Home Remedy Kit

Homeopathic remedies are derived from animal, vegetable, and mineral sources. Some of these sources, in their crude state, are highly toxic. *Belladonna* is made from a plant, deadly nightshade, that is accurately named; its red berries are poisonous. *Arsenicum album* is made from the metal arsenic, a deadly poison. Strange as it may seem, the most noxious substances make the most potent healing agents when prepared homeopathically.

As you may remember from our earlier discussion, the process of preparing homeopathic medicine, potentization (diluting and shaking, or grinding, the substance at each stage of dilution) produces a medicine that contains only trace amounts of the original substance. What is left is the medicinal essence of the substance, or what a physicist has called "energized medicine," so that all homeopathic medicines, regardless of their source, are harmless.

In the following introduction to the twenty-eight most frequently prescribed remedies, we have given the source of each remedy in parentheses. For a more complete description, see the *Meteria Medica* (Appendix C), which presents a "personality profile" of each remedy. The symptoms listed are those that provings of the remedy produced in healthy people. When these symptoms match your presenting symptoms, it is probable that particular medicine is your indicated remedy.

Do not expect to digest this information all at once. It is like meeting a roomful of people, in this case, all with foreign names; it takes time to sort them out. Throughout this book, we shall discuss these remedies—and many others—with their multiple characteristics over and over, so before long their Latin names will no longer sound strange and each will assume a distinct personality. As you gain experience in the use of these remedies, you will undoubtedly come to feel, as a member of a homeopathic study group expressed it, "The remedies are like old friends."

These are the medicines in the Home Remedy Kit:

Aconitum napellus (monkshood). *Aconite* is useful in the early stages of inflammation or fever and is indicated by the sudden onset of violent symptoms, especially after exposure to dry, cold wind. The patient who needs *Aconite* is fearful, restless, and thirsty for cold drinks.

Allium cepa (red onion). This remedy will help the person with a beginning cold who looks as if he has been peeling onions. There is frequent sneezing and the eyes stream; a watery discharge irritates the nose. The person may also have laryngitis, with a raw sensation extending into the chest.

Antimonium tartaricum (tartar emetic). *Antimonium tart* will benefit the person who has bronchitis and a wheezing cough; mucus in the chest makes a rattling bubbling sound as if the patient were drowning in his own secretions. He or she is pale, has a cold sweat, and looks sick.

Apis mellifica (honeybee). This remedy will relieve insect bites, including bee stings, or other rosy red spots with stinging pains.

Arnica montana (leopard's bane). Your first thought for the after effects of a fall or over-exertion, or injury from a blunt object. The person who needs *Arnica* feels bruised and sore.

Arsenicum album (arsenic). This is the most frequently needed remedy for stomach upsets, vomiting, or diarrhea, especially when caused by food poisoning.

Belladonna (deadly nightshade) The *Belladonna* patient is flushed, hot, and restless; symptoms are violent, with the onset sudden. The person may have a sore throat or cough, headache, earache, or fever.

Bryonia alba (white bryonia). *Bryonia* is called the "grumpy bear" because the person who needs it is irritable and wants to be left alone. Whatever the ailment—fever, headache, sore throat, stomach upset—the patient feels worse from the slightest movement and is very thirsty.

Calcarea phosphorica (phosphate of lime). *Calcarea phos* aids in the healing of bones and is therefore prescribed for fractures and difficult teething. This remedy also has a beneficial effect on tonsils and neck glands and on school children's headaches.

Cantharis (Spanish fly). *Cantharis* relieves the frequent, painful urination that occurs in cystitis. It also alleviates the pain of burns and scalds.

Carbo vegetabilis (vegetable charcoal). *Carbo veg.* is known as "the great reviver": it helps the person who is on the verge of collapse or whose vitality is low after an illness.

Chamomilla (German chamomile). The *Chamomilla* child when teething is irritable and cranky and just plain "impossible." *Chamomilla* is helpful for anyone who is oversensitive to pain, particularly when suffering from a toothache.

Ferrum phosphoricum (phosphate of iron). *Ferrum phos.* helps in the early stages of all inflammatory problems, including head colds, earache, cough, pneumonia, bronchitis, pleurisy, and rheumatism.

Gelsemium sempervirens (yellow jasmine). A remedy to consider if the person feels dull, heavy-lidded, complains of aching and chills, is not thirsty and wants to be left alone. *Gelesmium* is often needed for flu, head colds, tension headache.

Hepar sulphuris calcareum (calcium sulphide). *Hepar sulph.* helps to localize inflammation, as in bringing a boil to a head. It is useful for certain types of head colds, sore throat, laryngitis, and is the most frequently used remedy for children with croup.

Hypericum perfoliatum (St. John's wort). We call this the "*Arnica* of the nerves" because *Hypericum* heals injured parts rich in nerves, such as fingertips and toes. It also helps tailbone injuries, even old ones.

Ignatia amara (St. Ignatius bean). *Ignatia* is the grief remedy for the person who doesn't recover from an emotional upset such as disappointment or anger; patient sighs very frequently.

Ipecacuanha (ipecac root). *Ipecac* relieves constant nausea with or without vomiting. It also helps to stop a bad nosebleed or bleeding from any part of the body.

Ledum palustre (marsh tea). This is the key remedy for puncture wounds, stings, and bites. *Ledum* is also helpful in eye injuries and in sprained ankle.

Magnesia phosphorica (phosphate of magnesia). Some people call this the "homeopathic aspirin." *Magnesia phos.* eases any spasmodic pain that is relieved by warmth, such as leg cramp, menstrual cramps, or colic.

Mercurius vivus (quicksilver). This remedy is often indicated for tonsillitis, abscessed ears, boils, and gum disease. The person who needs *mercury* is sweaty, feels weak and trembling, and is very sensitive to temperature changes.

Nux vomica (poison nut). *Nux* is sometimes called the "hangover remedy" because it often relieves the person who has overindulged in food or alcohol. It also helps the chronic user of laxatives to break the habit.

Phosphorus (phosphorus). Some of the symptoms that indicate a need for *phosphorus* are laryngitis, a chest cold, hemorrhaging. *Phosphorus* has a long-lasting effect and should not be repeated often.

Pulsatilla (wind flower). This remedy will help a "ripe" cold with profuse thick yellowish discharge. It will also relieve the person who has an upset stomach from eating too much rich food. The person who needs *Pulsatilla* loves the open air, is worse from warmth, is not thirsty, and can't stand fat.

Ruta graveolens (rue). For a shinbone injury, or any injury to the periosteum (bone covering). It is also useful for sprains. When *Arnica* fails to relieve a bruised, lame feeling resulting from a fall, follow up with *Ruta*.

Spongia tosta (roasted sponge). This remedy's chief symptom is a croupy, wheezing cough, and therefore it is often prescribed for children during an attack of croup.

Sulphur (sublimated sulphur). Homeopaths often prescribe this medication for certain skin diseases that cause dry, itchy skin. *Sulphur* is more often used in chronic diseases than acute ones.

Veratrum album (white hellebore). A remedy for the distressful time when diarrhea and vomiting occur simultaneously. The patient is in a cold sweat, and feels faint.

The remedies in the homeopathic household kit are 6x potency. "Potency" refers to the number of times that a homeopathic remedy is diluted and succussed (shaken) or triturated (ground). Potency is indicated by one x for each time the process of dilution and succussion (or trituration) has been repeated. Thus "6x" on the label means that the entire process has been repeated six times. To help you better understand the meaning of potency, here is a brief description of the way in which a homeopathic remedy is prepared. Except for the use of machines, the process has not changed since Hahnemann's time.

In preparing *Arnica*, for example, which is extracted from a plant known as leopard's bane, the homeopathic pharmacist dissolves one part of the plant extract, or mother tincture with nine parts of the water/alcohol mixture and vigorously shakes (succusses) the mixture ten times, striking it with rhythmic sharp downward blows. The result is a 1x potency. When one part of this first dilution is mixed with nine parts of a fresh alcohol/water solution, again succussed ten times, the result is a 2x potency. Continuing this process to the sixth dilution, each time with nine parts of diluent, produces the 6x potency, as provided in our kit.

If the remedy to be potentized is insoluble in water, as for example, *Mercurius*, the pharmacist grinds the substance to the finest powder, a process called trituration, then mixes one part of this fine powder with nine parts of lactose (milk sugar), and grinds for an hour in a cleanmortar to produce the 1x potency. Repeating the process with fresh lactose produce the 2x potency; another repetition produce the 3x and so on to the 6x potency we seek.

Higher potencies, because they have proven to be more powerful and deeper acting than lower potencies, should be prescribed only by a physician. The decision as to which potency to prescribe is a complex one and requires many years of study and clinical experience on the part of the homeopathic physician.

You can safely treat your acute ailments with a well-chosen 6x potency, but if you are under the care of a homeopathic physician, you should not treat an acute condition with a remedy without the approval of your doctor. Oftentimes, an ailment that appears to be an acute condition may actually be caused by a deep acting remedy "working itself out." If so, taking a 6x potency could disorder the entire case and spoil the efforts of a physician and patient. Don't underestimate the effect of 6x potency; if it is the correct remedy, its action can be very powerful.

When and How to Use Your Kit

If you're the new owner of a household kit, you may be anxious to try it out, and therefore imagine you need a remedy for an inconsequential ailment. Resist this tendency; your kit is not a candy box for sampling. It is not only unnecessary but unwise always to be taking something. A homeopathic remedy is a nontoxic substance that has no direct effect upon the body, but when the prescription is accurate enough to stimulate the defense mechanism, the remedy is capable of disrupting the orderly functioning of that defense mechanism. **Have faith in your body. If you're reasonably healthy, your defense mechanism can shake off a minor ailment if given a chance.** So, unless this ailment is making you very uncomfortable. don't interfere with your body's curative powers by taking medicine— whether it's a pain killer, tranquilizer, or a homeopathic remedy.

Homeopathic remedies are easy to give and they act rapidly, but they must be used in accordance with the principles of the art discussed in chapter 1. These are

* **The law of similars**. Match the symptoms of the patient as closely as possible to the symptoms that were produced in healthy human beings when the medicine was proved.

* **The single remedy.** Give only one remedy at a time. Each substance is specific to a

certain set of disease symptoms; giving two or more remedies at a time introduces unknown elements into the picture: Which medication is causing what effect and how are they interacting?

* **The minimum dose.** This does not refer to the size of the dose but denotes the degree of potentization (6x) in the homeopathically prepared remedy, as explained earlier in this chapter.

The Dosage

The standard dosage in acute ailments is two tablets of the 6x every two to four hours. In chapter 4, "Accidents," we have recommended external remedies which are best used in the form of lotions. To prepare a lotion, simply dissolve one-half teaspoon tincture in one cup clean water and apply directly to the affected area.

"Standard dosage" notwithstanding, each case is individual. The interval between doses relates directly to the urgency of the situation, as in an acutely painful condition such as an earache requiring a dose every fifteen minutes. If there is no relief within an hour, you have probably chosen the wrong remedy and need to reassess the case. Homeopathy requires intelligence, careful observation, and common sense; otherwise, you would be reading the label on a bottle instead of this book!

Continue giving a remedy until improvement starts, then increase the interval between doses; when improvement is well established, discontinue the remedy. Imagine that you are pushing someone on a swing; you give only enough pushes to keep the swing going. Each dose is a push; if you push at the wrong time you may not stop the swinging, but you will interfere with the happy rhythmic motion. Some cases are more clear-cut than others, but if you keep a careful record of the patient's symptoms, you will probably sense when the person is on the mend, or needs another remedy. Prolonged use of a remedy, beyond the time when it is needed, may result in a backlash, or "aggravation"; that is, the patient "proves" the remedy and develops symptoms, as did the test subjects who first took the remedy to find out what it could do.

How to Take A Remedy

To take a remedy, tip the dose onto your clean palm or onto a spoon, and transfer to the tongue. If you are giving the dose to someone else, use his or her palm rather than yours. If you inadvertently pour out more tablets or granules than needed for the dose, discard the excess; do not replace them in the bottle because you may contaminate the remainder of your medicine. When opening the bottle, make certain that nothing touches the inside portion of the cork or cap, and close the bottle as soon as possible. Never have more than one of the remedies open at the same time as contamination can take place through airborne particles.

Medicine should be taken in a clean mouth. By "clean" we mean free of food, drink, tobacco, smoke, toothpaste, mouthwash, mints, or any matter except plain water. It is best not to wash down the dose with water: allow it to be absorbed directly through the mucous membrane of the mouth. The best time for taking a remedy is in the morning before breakfast and before brushing the teeth. Put nothing in the mouth except water fifteen minutes before or after the dose.

While taking a homeopathic medicine, avoid all other medicines such as aspirin, laxatives, sleeping pills, and patent medicines of any kind. Do not use nasal drops, antiseptics, liniments, or preparations containing camphor such as Chapstick. Saline mouthwash and *Calendula* antiseptic make good substitutes and will not interfere with homeopathic treatment. Eliminate coffee, which may neutralize the action of the homeopathic remedy.

Storage

Homeopathic remedies have indefinite shelf life if handled and stored properly. Always keep medicines in the container in which they were supplied; never transfer them to another bottle. This is a good habit to cultivate, as we are dealing with such minute quantities that trace elements of matter, which can cling to the interior of a bottle, may contaminate the fresh supply.

Keep medicines away from strong light, heat, and pungent odors such as camphor, menthol, mothballs, carbolic soap, and perfume. As an added protection, place your kit in an outer container. If your closet smells of mothballs, a locked bureau drawer is a good storage place. Keep out of reach of small children. A homeopathic remedy, even an entire vial consumed at one gulp, is not toxic or poisonous, but a toddler, intent on sampling the sweet-tasting pills, can wreak havoc on your kit.

OBSERVATION: THE KEY TO PRESCRIBING

The essence of homeopathy is building resistance, or stimulating the body's defense mechanism by selecting a remedy whose characteristics or "drug picture" matches the totality of the symptoms. The key to the choice of remedy is provided by the observation of those small differences that distinguish one person from another.

Two people "bitten" by the same bug may react differently, and therefore require different remedies. Take, for example, Jane and Dick, a couple who were exposed to a streptococcus infection at a party. Both became ill shortly after. Jane was flushed, restless, burning with heat, thirstless, and acutely ill all of a sudden. Her throat was bright red, and her head pounded with each strong pulsebeat. Jane needed *Belladonna* (deadly nightshade) for the strep infection. She took it and subsequently recovered rapidly.

Dick was not so quick to show symptoms. He gradually became quieter, grew pale, and was very thirsty for large drinks of cold water, and wanted to lie perfectly still and be let alone; he was extremely irritable when questioned or disturbed. He developed a dry, racking cough. Dick needed *Bryonia* (white bryon), and, after taking a dose, felt better, apologized for his irritability, and was soon over his illness and back to work with no after effects.

If each had taken the other's remedy, that is, if Jane had taken *Bryonia* and Dick *Belladonna*—a highly unlikely situation because no homeopathic prescriber, even a beginner, could mistake these two remedy pictures—the "wrong" remedy would probably have had no effect at all. Jane and Dick might each have concluded, "I've tried homeopathy and it doesn't work." This kind of reaction to homeopathy occurs frequently; someone is treated with a homeopathically *prepared* substance that was not homeopathically *applied*, and, predictably, "nothing happens."

There is no such thing as an innately "homeopathic remedy." A remedy is homeopathic *only* when it is given for a condition whose symptoms match the symptoms of the "remedy

YOUR HOME REMEDY KIT

picture," that is, the symptoms produced by the remedy when "proven" by a healthy subject. A wrong remedy is never homeopathic to the illness. Only the remedy which is homeopathic to the illness can produce the desired result.

To be a good prescriber, that is, to find the remedy to match the symptoms of the ill person, you must be alert for those individual symptoms we call "rare and peculiar." You can train yourself to be a good observer by learning what to observe. If you've taken care of a small child, then you have already learned to be aware of the nonverbal expressions that signify discomfort, likes, and dislikes. An ill person of any age may not feel like making the effort to answer questions, so use your eyes, ears, nose, your sense of touch—observe!

Here is an Observation Checklist for the home prescriber. Knowing what to look for will make it easier or match the symptoms of the patient to the remedy. After you've used this Observation Checklist a few times, the process will become almost second nature.

Before attempting to prescribe, use all your senses and observe:

Color of skin—Is it pale, red, or circumscribed red?
Color of lips—Are they red or pale, dry or cracked?
Color of tongue—Is it red-tipped, red-streaked, white, or swollen? Is it dry or wet?
Expression—Is it anxious, frightened, stupefied, confused? Do the eyelids droop?
Position and movement—Is the patient quiet and still, lethargic or restless?
Mood—Is the patient irritable, nervous, angry, sad, or withdrawn?
State of mind—Is the patient irrational or delirious?
Skin—Is it dry, moist, clammy, hot, cool or cold, sensitive to touch?
Pulse—Is it rapid, slow, weak, or pounding?
How does the patient respond to touch—Does it hurt or comfort him?
Voice—Is it weak, hoarse, deep or husky?
Breathing—Is it gasping, rapid, difficult, wheezing, or irregular?
Speech—Is it incoherent, rushed, slow, or does the patient refuse to answer?
Where does it hurt? Determine the precise location of the pain. Ask the patient to point to painful spot with one finger.
At what time does the patient feel worse—morning, noon, afternoon, evening, or night? Before or after midnight?
What kind of pain is the patient experiencing? Is it aching, boring, bruised, burning or bursting, cramping, cutting or dull? Is the pain like a nail being driven in, or is it pressing or stitching?
What are the patient's physical wants? Does he crave fresh air? Does he ask for cold or hot drinks? Does he like cold applications or warm ones? Does he feel better in general from warmth or from cold?
How does he smell—sick, sour, sweet, musty, or offensive?

For example, your husband, Jack, comes home complaining of a headache and doesn't want any dinner. He goes to bed at once and asks for an extra blanket. He had seemed fine when he left this morning, but now his temperature registers 102 degrees fahrenheit; he is chilly, beginning to ache all over, and can't seem to get warm. When you look in on him, he appears to be asleep but, on closer look, you see he is awake with drooping eyelids. You offer him a drink of water that he refuses.

Making your observations according to the Observation Checklist, you note that his face appears flushed, with dry lips, and his expression dull and stupefied. He is quiet and lethargic and wants to be let alone. He becomes irritable only when you persist in questioning him. Touching him, you find his skin is hot and dry; although he complains of feeling chilly. He has a slightly sour or sickish odor. When you ask him about his headache, he replies in a weak voice that it's a dull aching pressure like a band around his head.

Turning to chapter 7, "How to Prevent and Treat Colds, Coughs, and Earaches," you note that Jack's symptoms correspond to the symptoms of *Gelsemium* (yellow jasmine) as listed in the chapter summary. *Gelsemium*'s "guiding symptoms" include: "drowsy, sluggish, chilly, tiredness and aching of whole body, headache, mild fever, lack of thirst . . . ." Other remedies such as *Arsenicum* (arsenic) and *Bryonia* have one or two of the same symptoms, but only *Gelsemium* matches all of the patient's symptoms.

Sometimes a remedy picture is not that clear-cut. If so, turn to the Mini-Repertory (Appendix B) and follow the directions. Used in conjunction with the *Materia Medica* (Appendix C) and the remedy summaries that appear at the end of each chapter, the Mini-Repertory will help you become adept in the use of homeopathic remedies at home. As you will discover, it is both an art and a science.

Even given the right remedy, speed of recovery will vary from person to person. Jack may recover overnight, provided that he has a strong defense mechanism, or what we call a "good constitution." On the other hand, he may not be so fortunate. Perhaps he has inherited a tendency toward diabetes and his health is further affected by living in a city that has a high pollution index. In addition, he works in an office in which several people smoke, further polluting his air space. Under these circumstances, Jack may take several days to recover, but he will do so in less time than he would if he dosed himself with patent medicines that suppress symptoms rather than assist the defense mechanism.

Make a habit of keeping a notebook in which you jot down symptoms of each family member during an illness. Besides helping you as a prescriber, the notebook will serve as a record of the course of the illness and, over a period of time, show the patterns of illness in the family and the most successful prescriptions.

If you live alone or are the only member of the family trained in homeopathy, it is wise to familiarize yourself with the remedies and their indications while you're alert and well. In the event that you become acutely ill, if possible, write down all your symptoms. This will make it easier for you to be objective about your condition. Although it's nice to be looked after when you're sick, as a prescriber you have the advantage of knowing better than anyone else how you feel.

THE COMBINATION GAME

One last word about remedies. You may have seen advertisements for combination tablets for specific acute ailments. The appeal of the combinations is understandable; they bypass the problem of individualizing the prescription to match the remedy to the patient. An English naturopath, Eric F. W. Powell, writes: "It is an extremely difficult matter to find the correct remedy in the majority of cases. . . . By combining several remedies. . . the resulting cures were often beyond all expectation."

An article about combination remedies, published by Standard Homeopathic Company of Los Angeles, predicts: "More and more practitioners will learn to use these combination forms, not as a substitute for the single remedy, but as a valuable tool in instances where it is just not feasible to fully repertorize a patient."

This is a controversial issue among homeopathic physicians. There is no question that a combination remedy designed for a specific acute condition is a time-saver, and, on rare occasions, I have prescribed one. But many of us believe that far better results are obtained in the long run by adhering strictly to fundamental laws of homeopathy, which include the single remedy.

In this chapter, you have become acquainted with the twenty-eight remedies in the homeopathic household kit. It's comforting to know that you're prepared for a sudden illness or emergency, but don't imagine you need a remedy because "it's there." It is important to realize that the least medicine is the best medicine. One of my long-time patients said to me, "I use less and less medicine, each year." She has learned respect for the power of the homeopathic remedy as well as for the ability of the defense mechanism to cope without medicine.

4

What to Do for Accidents

NOTHING can make you more conscious of the value of homeopathy than reading a standard text on first aid. "Elevate the limb. . . . Apply ice, then heat. . . ." All good commonsense measures, but homeopathy can do so much more to relieve pain and promote healing, as you will discover in this chapter.

In dealing with the various conditions classified as "accidents"—bruises, sprains and strains, wounds, insect stings and bites, burns, and sports injuries—you will need the following internal remedies: *Apis mellifica*, *Arnica montana*, *Bryonia alba*, *Cantharis*, *Hepar sulphuris*, *Hypericum*, *Ledum palustre*, *Phosphorus*, *Rhus toxicodendron*,* *Ruta graveolens*, *Symphytum officinale*.*

Among the most useful preparations for external use are *Arnica* tincture, *Calendula officinalis succus* (a liquid preparation containing minimal alcohol), *Calendula* ointment, *Hypericum* tincture, *Ledum* tincture, and *Urtica urens* tincture.

In general, internal remedies seem to be more effective than external, but when your child scrapes a knee or your spouse gets a finger crushed, it's comforting to apply a lotion made from one of the tinctures. In the end-of-chapter summary table, remedies are grouped under their specific accident category so that you can see the alternatives at a glance. Use whichever one you have on hand. (In the following chapters, choosing a remedy involves more subtle distinctions; the remedies will therefore be listed by themselves.)

BRUISES (CONTUSIONS)

A bruise is an injury caused by a blow from a blunt object which damages the soft tissues beneath the skin. For example, when you hit yourself with a hammer or fall downstairs, this injury crushes the innumerable tiny blood vessels that form a network throughout your body, releasing blood into the tissues. The injury turns blue and purple and eventually yellow, and then disappears. The medical term for bruise is contusion.

Your first thought in treating a bruise should be *Arnica*. *Arnica montana* is made from a plant called leopard's bane that grows in the mountains. Its name in German is "fall-kraut"; peasants observed that if a sheep or goat fell down a hillside and hurt itself, it

---

*Not included in Home Remedy Kit.

would nibble the leaves of this plant.

Hahnemann, who founded homeopathy in the early 1800s, was the first to test *Arnica* scientifically. While "proving" the remedy, Hahnemann and several colleagues reported a bruised feeling all over, an aching back as if after a bad fall, the sensation of shock. According to the law of similars, the symptoms that *Arnica* produces in healthy people are the symptoms that *Arnica* can cure.

Take two tablets of *Arnica* every three to four hours; place dry on the tongue and dissolve in the mouth. Discontinue medicine as soon as improvement is noted. When pain is intense, take *Arnica* every fifteen minutes until pain subsides. Frequency of dosage depends on the severity of pain, so act accordingly. As an added aid, apply *Arnica* externally to the bruised area like rubbing alcohol, but do not use when the skin is broken as it will irritate the skin.

My most memorable experience with *Arnica* was during my medical days at Ohio State University, when I had a room in a friendly boarding house with uncarpeted stairs. One night I started down the stairs. I was wearing slippers, and suddenly my feet went out from under me. I grabbed the banister, which, instead of saving me, came along with me! I fell back on my head and spine. I was conscious of a tightness in my chest and a blurring of vision from shock.

Arnica has the ability to counteract the effect of shock that so often accompanies a fall or injury. So, after catching my breath, I crept back to my room and took two tablets of *Arnica*. The next morning, I apologized to my landlady for the damage to the banister, but she was more concerned about my condition. I had no bruises or black and blue marks, which surprised her.

A few weeks later, my lab partner, a woman twenty years my junior, had a similar fall, and was bruised and sore for days. She couldn't understand why I, at my advanced age, had escaped unscathed. I regret that I didn't have the courage to tell her about *Arnica*, not wanting to be labeled an oddball in that stronghold of orthodox medicine.

Other homeopaths develop the same affection for *Arnica*. I was talking to a young family practitioner, Dr. David C. Fabrey of Cincinnati, who told me that he was surprised and pleased to find that homeopathic remedies really worked. Shortly after obtaining his kit of remedies, he moved into a new apartment. "I was dragging my refrigerator when it fell on my leg—banged the knee, which turned red and began to swell. I took one dose of *Arnica*, and within one hour all the soreness was gone."

My patients regard *Arnica* as a trusted friend and usually have it with them at all times. Recently, I attended a meeting of our local homeopathic study group. After the meeting, one of the members tripped and fell in the parking lot. As if on cue, several of her classmates rushed over and fished out *Arnica* from handbags or coat pockets.

Although *Arnica* is helpful in all types of bruises, certain injuries will respond better to *Hypericum*, known as "the *Arnica* of the nerves." If you should catch your finger in a car door, fall on your tailbone, have your toe crushed on a dance floor—any of these painful situations call for *Hypericum*. This remedy, made from a plant called St. John's wort, has special healing powers for parts rich in nerves such as fingertips, toes, spine, palms, or soles.

I discovered *Hypericum*'s healing powers when I was a small child and someone slammed a car door on my hand. This was at least fifty years ago, but I can still remember that it was my right fourth finger that took the brunt of that awful force and turned white. When I arrived home, my father, a homeopathic physician, quickly placed two tablets in my mouth, and the throbbing pain began to ease. Gently but firmly he reshaped the crushed finger, and it was fine after that.

Ledum is another remedy that acts on bruised nerves. *Ledum palustre*, sometimes called marsh tea, is made from a small shrub resembling a tea plant. Its white flowers contain an antiseptic camphorlike oil which smells somewhat like hops.

When a bruise persists longer than seems reasonable and the injured part remains cold and numb, this is an indication for *Ledum*. The keynote for *Ledum* in any problems is "relieved by cold." One day, Dr. James Tyler Kent, the renowned homeopath, was making a house call to see a patient suffering from excessively swollen hands and feet. The doctor found him sitting with his feet in a tub filled with ice water. A dose of *Ledum* relieved the patient of his need for ice-cold soaks and cured the swelling in his extremities. When a severe bruise remains swollen and discolored despite using *Arnica*, *Ledum* will often complete the healing. Think of *Ledum* when a bruise results in a black eye or "shiner."

A third remedy for specific types of bruises is *Ruta graveolens*. Rue, its common name, "the herb of grace," has been used as an herbal medicine for thousands of years. When the shinbone is bruised, this injures the sensitive bone covering known as the periosteum. *Ruta* acts specifically on these tissues, as well as on sprained wrists and ankles.

Recently, a patient told of tripping over a puppy's bed placed near the stairs to the basement and pitching headlong down the stairs. Grasping the edge of one step halfway down, she was fortunate to emerge with nothing worse than a badly scraped shin. "There was a red gash over the entire length of the shinbone that burned like fire," she said.

She took *Arnica* to ease the shock, then treated the wound with *Calendula* lotion and applied a sterile dressing. Next day, the bruised periosteum was excessively tender to the touch. She took a dose of *Ruta* and within a few hours the tenderness was gone.

Ruta, like most of our homeopathic remedies, has multiple uses, as you'll discover in our chapters on headaches and stomach and bowel problems.

BEYOND FIRST AID: If the victim has been struck on the head, observe him or her carefully for signs of head injury. Generally, a person is dazed or confused after a sudden injury, but if the dazed condition worsens, seek professional medical help.

A fall or blow may also injure internal organs as indicated by increased pulse rate, pale skin, increasing shock. If this condition persists for any length of time following an accident, seek professional help at once.

In these serious situations, give *Arnica* immediately. If patient is unconscious, soften two tablets in one-quarter teaspoon of water and place the tablets under the tongue or inside the cheek.

SPRAINS

A sprain is an injury to the soft tissue about a joint, causing muscles, ligaments, and tendons to be stretched or torn. A ligament is a band of fibrous tissue tying bones together. A tendon is a fibrous band that connects a muscle to a bone. The most common sprains are of the ankles, fingers, wrists, and knees.

Since shock is always present when a sprain occurs, give a dose of *Arnica* immediately. *Arnica* controls shock as well as bleeding in the tissues, and may be all that is needed. If, however, after a day or so improvement seems at a standstill, *Ruta graveolens* will help. *Ruta* acts on torn and wrenched tendons, ligaments, and also on the bruised periosteum, or bone coverings.

A patient, Virginia, a journalist, benefited from *Ruta* when she tripped and fell down some stone steps at the courthouse. "I was wearing a new pair of sling-back shoes and lost my balance," she said. "I went into shock and collapsed. I wished I'd had *Arnica* with me, but once I rested for a while, I was all right, except for a bad sprain." Once home, she elevated her leg and took a dose of *Ruta*. The next day, she limped a bit and the swelling gradually subsided. The following day, she wasn't conscious of her injury at all, she said.

If *Ruta* does not relieve the pain from torn connective tissue within twenty-four hours, take *Symphytum*, a deeper-acting remedy. *Symphytum* is made from the plant comfrey, which the ancient physicians called "knit-bone." You can take this "knit-bone" internally or apply *Symphytum* lotion as a dressing or ointment.

A colleague, Dr. Marion Belle Rood, told me how effective *Symphytum* was in treating a patient with a jump fracture. This is a type of fracture of the small bones of the foot which includes disruptions of tendons and ligaments. The patient fell from a high wall and landed on his feet, shattering one heel. Dr. Rood gave him *Symphytum* and reshaped the heel gently in her hands. She then applied a dressing of shaved thin slices of comfrey root, and bandaged it. Healing was prompt, and on the patient's next visit, his heel looked normal.

When a sprain causes joints to become hot, swollen, and painful, *Rhus toxicodendron*, made from the poison ivy plant, will help. *Rhus tox.* is often called the "rusty gate" remedy. A person who needs the remedy feels creaky on first movement and better when limbered up.

Rhus tox., like *Ruta*, is often a good remedy to follow *Arnica* after *Arnica* has done all it can. I experienced this on a recent trip to Greece. I was attending a seminar in Athens, and early in my visit wrenched my ankle severely on some uneven pavement. With the help of my companion, I limped back to the hotel and took *Arnica*. The next day, with an elastic bandage wrapped snugly around my ankle, I was able to walk to the lecture, a trek of a mile each way. In fact, my ankle felt better after I had walked a few blocks.

But after several days, the ankle didn't seem to be improving any further; it was swollen and discolored. So I took *Rhus tox.*, which has the strong symptom, "Feels better after moving." The remedy helped considerably; I was hardly aware of my injury after that.

Other homeopathic remedies to consider when treating sprains:

Bryonia. When the joint near the injury becomes swollen and distended and painful on the least movement.

Ledum. When there is much swelling, and the injured joint is cold and numb but feels better with cold application.

COMMONSENSE MEASURES: Elevate the injured part. Apply an ice bag or cold compress over the sprain to reduce swelling and pain. Apply *Arnica* lotion as a moist compress, and a firm bandage for support.

BEYOND FIRST AID: If the sprain seems severe, seek professional help. Meanwhile, take whichever remedy mentioned in this section most closely fits the symptoms.

STRAINS

A strain is a muscle injury in which muscle fibers are stretched and sometimes partially torn. A strain generally causes swelling and pain in the affected muscle.

Most common are those of the back muscles, usually caused by lifting. If the principal sensation is a sore, bruised feeling, *Arnica* is the remedy. The early spring days, when the ground is first workable, always brings a crop of weekend farmers into my waiting room.

Like the weekend athlete, these enthusiasts plunge into full activity without conditioning. *Arnica*, which is our chief remedy for sore muscles quickly relieves their distress.

For those who are worse when beginning to move but better after stirring around, *Rhus tox*. will be more helpful. *Rhus tox*. acts on the connective tissue covering the muscles, on torn ligaments, and tendons.

My secretary, Anne, tells me that back trouble is the most frequent complaint among the males in her family. Her husband works in construction and now and then strains his back lifting heavy materials. Anne's two older sons shovel coal for the same company, an activity that frequently causes back strain. After observing that each felt better after limbering up, Anne prescribed *Rhus tox*. and all three benefited from it. She also told them to rest as much as possible and use a heat pad.

BEYOND FIRST AID: If pain persists or worsens, seek professional help.

WOUNDS

A wound is a break in the skin, and often the soft tissues beneath the skin are damaged as well.

There are four types of wounds: incisions, lacerations, scratches and abrasions, and punctures. An incised wound is clean cut. A lacerated wound is torn, and may be jagged. An abrasion is a scrape which rubs off the top layer of skin. A puncture wound is made by a sharp object such as a nail, tack, or pin.

Calendula officinalis, prepared from the tall, wild marigold, "the herb of the sun," is the chief homeopathic medicine for wounds. The late Dorothy Shepherd, a British homeopath who had vast experience treating wounds as a medical officer at an outpatient center in London during World War II, describes *Calendula* as "the most satisfactory wound dressing I have come across. . . [It] is not an antiseptic in the true meaning of the word, but germs do not thrive in its presence. It inhibits their growth, I find, and even when wounds are already badly infected, I have seen offensive purulent discharges become clean and sweet smelling in a day or two."

A New York surgeon, Dr. Edmund Carlton, who practiced in the early 1900s, extolled the virtues of *Calendula*. In his book, *Homeopathy in Medicine and Surgery*, he writes. "I would almost as soon leave my instruments at home when going out to cut as my *Succus calendulae*. No antisepsis is allowed to interfere with the practice . . . That well-nigh universal fetish (poisoning of wound and system with drugs) has never received my worship."

Until ten or fifteen years ago, surgeons scrubbing before an operation dipped their hands in iodine or alcohol and painted a form of iodine on the patient's skin. Today, surgeons have discontinued using these strong antiseptics, realizing that they are very irritating to the tissues and inhibit healing. So, we may hope that as homeopathy becomes better known, an adventurous surgeon will do as Dr. Carleton did, and use *Calendula* in the operating room.

Homeopaths have always depended on *Calendula* as a first-aid measure. When my daughter Della was in second grade, her favorite stunt on a winter day while wearing slippery ski pants was to run over the oiled classroom floor and land on her knees. One day, a splinter ran through her pants and became imbedded in her knee, like an arrow. Not being a doctor at the time, I took her to a kindly neighborhood physician who removed the splinter and applied an antiseptic. Having been raised in a homeopathic family, I promptly washed off the antiseptic when we got home and applied *Calendula*. The puncture wound healed quickly with no infection.

Calendula is not the only external wound remedy. *Hypericum* and *Ledum* are also useful in treating wounds, and each has its special attribute. *Hypericum* lotion is particularly effective in relieving pain of injured nerves. *Ledum* lotion is helpful for puncture wounds and sprains.

Note that *Arnica*, our old standby, is missing from this list of external wound remedies. Never apply *Arnica* tincture or lotion to an open wound; it will usually irritate the skin severely.

I discovered this, much to my sorrow, when my daughter Anne, as a little girl, got a nasty cut on her hand when a glass broke as she was washing dishes. I cleaned it up; then, in my ignorance, I applied *Arnica* lotion. The cut healed but blisterlike eruptions developed around the edge of the wound. They subsided slowly during the course of a week.

Incised Wound

To treat a superficial incised wound, cleanse with *Hypericum* or *Calendula* lotion, apply a sterile gauze dressing and bandage, and leave the dressing undisturbed. (A dressing is the material that you put directly over the wound; a bandage holds the dressing in place.) Keep dressing moist by dabbing on *Calendula* or *Hypericum* lotion the first day or so, but do not remove the dressing, even though it is bloodstained and becomes smelly. Change the bandage or add to the dressing if need be, but do not change the dressing covering the wound.

Sometimes, in spite of good care, the wound becomes inflamed. You will know this from the way it feels: the bandage may seem tight owing to swelling, and you may see red extending beyond the edge of the bandage. If this happens, take *Hepar sulphuris* three times a day for a few days. *Hepar sulph.* is a white powder from calcified oyster shells burned in a crucible with pure powdered sulphur.

COMMONSENSE MEASURES: Although healing usually proceeds rapidly with use of homeopathic treatment, many people find it helpful to take increased amounts of vitamins C, A, and E.

BEYOND FIRST AID: If an incised wound in the hand or foot is deep, and there is a possibility of a cut tendon, seek medical help at once.

Lacerated Wound

For a minor laceration, cleanse with mild soap and water, and apply a dressing moistened with *Calendula* lotion or *Hypericum* lotion. Bandage the dressing in place.

BEYOND FIRST AID: If laceration is extensive, *Arnica* may be needed for shock, and a clean dressing moistened with *Hypericum* lotion should be applied. Seek professional help at once. After the wound has been treated by a doctor, give *Hypericum* internally three times a day; or, if the pain is very great, give hourly until better. Later, stop *Hypericum* and give *Arnica* two or three times a day to speed healing.

Scratches and Abrasions

These can be extremely painful and dangerous if the raw skin is contaminated with dirt or other foreign matter. Do not use any strong substance, such as iodine, that can burn the skin or irritate the delicate exposed tissues. When the epithelium, your protective shell, has been rubbed off, anything you put on the wound will be readily absorbed and can injure those delicate cells whose protective covering has been removed. Clean the area gently but thoroughly with *Calendula* lotion.

If you're over twenty-five, you probably grew up having your cuts and scrapes treated with tincture of iodine. You're not likely to forget it—the pungent smell, the searing pain as the applicator touched your raw skin. Or, you may have vivid memories of using iodine on your child's cuts. Undoubtedly, you felt as so many other people did, "This hurts me more than it hurts you!"

Iodine was once a staple item in every school and home first-aid kit. The 1925 edition of the *American Red Cross Abridged Textbook on First Aid* advises: "Painting iodine on wounds is unquestionably of considerable value in preventing their infection. The more promptly it is applied, the better."

A Seattle physician, Dr. Harry H. Kretzler, Sr., recalls rejecting this advice when teaching a Red Cross class in First Aid in the 1930s. "I taught my students to cleanse a wound with mild soap and water," Dr. Kretzler said, "but was informed by the Red Cross that my students would not pass the course if they failed to mention iodine in their exams."

Fifty years later, we scarcely hear about iodine. The authors of a popular family health guide, published in 1976, write: "All wounds should be washed with soap and water or a mild antiseptic solution." One reason for the decline of iodine was the observation that alcohol in solution tends to evaporate, leaving a more concentrated solution. As a result, many users of iodine suffer chemical burns.

BEYOND FIRST AID: If foreign matter is ingrained in the wound, treatment should be performed by a physician.

Puncture Wounds

Gently press around the wound to encourage bleeding. (Punctures tend to "seal in" contamination.) If the wound should bleed excessively, apply a clean dressing with slight pressure. After washing your hands thoroughly, check to make sure that no foreign object is left in the wound.

Ledum is the best remedy for puncture wounds; it prevents sepsis (disease germs in the blood and tissues) and promotes healing. Wash the cut with *Ledum* lotion, then soak the wound in water to which you have added a few drops of *Ledum*. Or, if not a soakable part, use a compress moistened with *Ledum* lotion. Do not use a swab in a puncture wound

WHAT TO DO FOR ACCIDENTS

because you do not want to damage more tissue. Soaking is best; you are trying to remove the surface dirt.

BEYOND FIRST AID: The danger in a puncture wound is tetanus. The germ is carried in by the nail, rusty or not, or whatever instrument caused the injury, and then thrives in the airless tract. Owing to the danger of tetanus, for any but the most minor puncture wound, seek professional help.

INSECT STINGS AND BITES

Bees, Hornets, and Wasps

These are among the most common insect stings. Immediately following an insect sting, one experiences a violent burning pain followed by itching and redness at the site. Sometimes a welt like a hive appears and then gradually subsides over the next few hours.

One of the most widely used homeopathic remedies for bee stings is *Apis mellifica*. *Apis* is made from the whole honey bee. Long before *Apis* was "proved," American Indians knew the healing properties of the honey bee. A physician in 1847 described how an Indian woman, a member of the Narragansett tribe, prepared the medicine from the crude bees. "She enclosed the bees in a covered tin pail, and placed them in a heated oven until they were killed, and then after powdering them, administered one in syrup every night and morning."

As described in the *U.S. Homeopathic Pharmacopoeia*, the live bees are now placed in a clean wide-mouthed stoppered bottle, which is shaken to irritate the bees. A mixture of glycerine, distilled water, and alcohol is poured into the bottle, and the bees soak in this mixture for ten days. The internal remedy is made from dilutions of this tincture.

Apis symptoms are: burning stinging pains, a rosy swelling rather than bright red, puffiness rather than firm, hard swelling, and worse from heat. This combination of symptoms indicates a need for *Apis*, whether the problem is a bee sting or edema from a kidney ailment.

It's not necessary to take an internal remedy every time you get a bee sting. Our feeling is, the less medicine, the better. But if the affected area is a knuckle or thumb—a part that allows little room for swelling—the sting can be extremely painful, and you'll welcome the relief that the indicated remedy will bring.

Unless the bee sting is really severe, an external remedy such as *Ledum* tincture will suffice. Take a cotton applicator and apply a drop or two of tincture. There's no need to prepare lotion. You need only a small amount, and, besides, the concentrated alcohol in the tincture may in itself have an antidotal effect on the venom.

If you don't have *Ledum* tincture on hand, substitute *Arnica, Calendula, Urtica urens* or *Hypericum* tincture.

These tinctures work rapidly as I observed last summer when Virginia, a houseguest, was stung by a wasp. The sting became very tender and annoying, so I brought out my bottle of *Ledum* tincture and dabbed on a drop or two. I went out of the room to put the bottle back and, when I returned, Virginia greeted me happily with the announcement that the tenderness was gone. There was only a faint redness to indicate the site of attack.

According to the Food and Drug Administration, an estimated thirty to fifty

Americans die annually from systemic reactions to insect stings, and approximately 1 to 2 million patients are at risk because of severe allergic reaction to stinging insects. If you or a member of your family is hypersensitive to bee stings, it would be wise to consult a homeopathic physician about obtaining high-potency *Apis*. A patient who used to suffer an allergic reaction, characterized by shortness of breath, anxiety, and a sensation of swelling of the throat, always carries a small packet of *Apis* to be taken immediately in case of bee stings. This helps, even though the ideal way to treat sensitivity to bee sting is constitutional prescribing.

If a bee sting does not produce *Apis* symptoms, there are other homeopathic remedies that are useful. As you may recall, *Ledum* heals puncture wounds, so it's not surprising that it frequently relieves a bee sting, which is a form of puncture wound. *Ledum* symptoms are numbness or sensitivity to touch and pains that may extend upward, relieved by cold.

Even before I became a physician, my first experience with *Ledum* convinced me that homeopathic remedies really work. My daughter Della, then five years old, was an adventurous child, and one day decided to investigate a buggy abandoned in a field near our house. Yellow jackets had built a nest there. Della climbed into the buggy, and the wasps descended on her. She came running to me, shrieking with pain, her face grotesquely swollen. I called our homeopathic physican, who advised *Ledum*, and told me to repeat the medicine when needed.

With the first dose, swelling subsided. Sitting by her bed side, I could see the swelling begin to return, the spots like hives where each bite had become white and was surrounded by a raised red area. Soon afterward, she became restless, stirred, then awakened and cried. I put another tablet of *Ledum* under her tongue, and soon she quieted down and went to sleep and the spots faded out. Later, during the night, the swelling would commence again, and I would repeat the dose. I gave her about eight doses before the swelling subsided for good.

If the affected part is red and inflamed looking and imparts a burning sensation, *Cantharis*, made from the Spanish Fly, may be the best choice. If severe pain radiates upward from the injury, this may indicate nerve involvement. If so, *Hypericum* will relieve it.

BEYOND FIRST AID: If the victim is allergic to insect stings, rush the person to the nearest hospital emergency room. Meanwhile, give *Apis* in the highest potency you have.

Poisonous Spiders, Scorpions, and Snakes

Common varieties of poisonous spiders and scorpions are the black widow spider, brown recluse spider, scorpion, and the U.S. tarantula. The four types of poisonous snakes in the U.S. are the rattlesnake, copperhead, moccasin, and coral snake. Their bite or sting is not always a matter of life or death, but does demand immediate action. There may be redness and swelling around the bite or sting, along with painful abdominal or muscle cramps, fever, sweating, and nausea. A tingling or burning pain may spread throughout the body.

These remedies are recommended if you should be bitten by a poisonous spider, scorpion, or snake.

Carbolicum acidum (carbolic acid). A patient needing this remedy has a dusky red face, is pale around the mouth and nose. Seems languid but has an increased awareness of odors.

Crotalus horridus (rattlesnake venom). Used in serious cases where symptoms rapidly follow bite of insect or snake. There is much swelling and discoloration around the bite.

Echinacea (purple cone flower, or thistle). Provings have not brought out clear indications, but this remedy has proved effective in blood poisoning and infection.

Lachesis (snake venom). Affected part is dusky red or blue; there may be oozing of dark blood.

Oxalicum acidum (oxalic acid). This remedy has proved valuable where the affected part is cold and numb, with violent pains and trembling.

If you're planning to backpack or live in an area infested with these venomous creatures, it would be wise for you to obtain the preparations mentioned above.

BEYOND FIRST AID: Apply an ice pack to the bite to slow the spread of the poison, and then rush the victim to the nearest hospital emergency room. Meanwhile, give one of the remedies mentioned above.

BURNS

Burns range from insignificant although painful injuries to life-threatening ones. The extent of body surface affected is a key to the seriousness of the injury. Burns that involve 10 percent of the total body surface, are considered minor, major burns cover more than 10 percent of the total body surface. (The surface area of the hand represents 1 per cent of the total body surface.)

In any burn there is the element of shock. Give *Arnica* immediately. One dose usually is enough; if shock persists, repeat as needed. After shock has passed, the burned person may feel more pain. If so, give *Cantharis* every fifteen minutes. Continue until improvement is noted. Repeat *Cantharis* if pain returns.

Women who live in farm country do a lot of canning, and inevitably some suffer burns or scalds. This happened to a patient, Martha, who received a steam scald on her right forearm that covered the entire arm from palm to elbow. When she called me, I told her to take *Cantharis*, two tablets every fifteen minutes for a few doses, then as the pain subsided, increase intervals between doses. I also recommended that she bathe her forearm with *Hypericum* lotion and then cover the burned area with a clean cloth moistened with the same lotion. When she came to the office the next morning, she said that the pain had stopped after the second dose of *Cantharis*, so she took no more. On examination, the arm showed no blisters; there was only pink skin with no breaks. The burned area healed swiftly without a scar.

I've had countless reports from patients on the effectiveness of *Cantharis*. Susan, a patient in Dayton, who is forever singeing herself while cooking, takes *Cantharis*. "Right away I can feel my burn cooling down," she said.

Causticum, a mineral preparation, is another effective internal remedy for burns. (We've mentioned *Cantharis* first because it is in your home remedy kit. Use whichever you have on hand). The late Dr. Dorothy Shepherd, author of *Homeopathy for the First-Aider*, used *Causticum* in severe cases of burning in which there was pain and restlessness along with blister formation. "The *Causticum* removes the agonies of the pain within seven to ten minutes and should be repeated whenever the pain returns."

Urtica urens tincture, made from the stinging nettle, is a soothing external burn remedy. It is best used in lotion form; one-half teaspoon of tincture in one cup of clean water. Pat on with sterile gauze, or apply compress moistened with *Urtica urens* lotion. *Hypericum* lotion and *Calendula* lotion are also external remedies for burns; use whichever you have on hand.

Kay, a patient who is well acquainted with homeopathic first-aid remedies, recalled the time her college-age daughter, Margo, received a coffee scald while working as a waitress. "Her entire chest was burned raw from the neck to the waist," Kay said. The burn was complicated by faulty treatment on the part of restaurant personnel; they had applied petroleum jelly to the burn and covered it with gauze. She was then sent to the emergency room where the petroleum jelly had to be removed, causing more pain and further injury to the tissues.

When Margo was brought home, Kay put her right to bed, gave her a dose of *Cantharis*, and called me. I told her to loosen the gauze with *Calendula* lotion (which acts as an antiseptic) and then to keep the burned area moist until the soreness was gone.

Kay kept a bowl of *Calendula* lotion at her daughter's bedside and dipped several large linen handkerchiefs into the lotion covering the burned area with them. For the next twenty-four hours, she kept the handkerchiefs saturated with lotion.

"Margo was so afraid she'd be scarred," Kay said, "but the burned area healed without the trace of a scar."

When I burn myself cooking, the first thing I do is cut a leaf from the *Aloe vera* plant that rests on the windowsill in my kitchen. The leaf of the plant, a tropical species, contains a slimy, jellylike substance. I split the leaf and rub its contents over the burn; the gel relieves pain by shutting out air, and has a healing effect. Incidentally, an *Aloe vera* plant requires little care and reproduces rapidly. The progeny of my original plant are flourishing in the kitchens of countless friends and patients.

COMMONSENSE MEASURES: Unwise first-aid treatment for burns can be extremely harmful. *Don't ever smear greasy ointment on the burn.* If the burn is severe, the doctor will have to remove the ointment, which subjects the victim to additional suffering.

Heat has already sterilized the burned area, and no unsterile material should be applied. To avoid contamination, cover with sterile gauze or a piece of clean cloth.

Immerse the burned area in cold water to which you have added a few drops of *Hypericum* or *Urtica urens* lotion. This relieves the pain and prevents pooling of fluid in the tissues around the burn.

If your clothing has been saturated with burning liquid, remove the garment immediately where it comes loose easily. If it sticks, cut around it. Wrap the area in a piece of clean material such as a sheet, towel, or washcloth.

Don't puncture blisters unless it's really necessary to relieve pain. A blister provides a sterile covering for the burn. When the blister is broken, the burn is open to infection.

An electrical burn is often more extensive than it looks because damage beneath the skin is apt to be greater than on the surface. Treat it as you would any severe burn.

WHAT TO DO FOR ACCIDENTS

Flush chemical burns copiously with water for at least five minutes; then treat as any other burn.

In the case of a severely burned patient, it's important to maintain fluid intake. If the victim is conscious, dissolve one teaspoon of salt in a pint of water. Give half a glass of this solution every fifteen minutes. Discontinue fluids if the patient vomits. Never try to make an unconscious person drink.

BEYOND FIRST AID: If a large surface of the body is burned, or if the burn is very deep, cover the victim with a clean sheet and rush him or her to the emergency room of the nearest hospital. Give *Arnica* immediately for shock.

SPORTS INJURIES

With the new emphasis on fitness, more and more people are jogging and playing tennis, racquet ball, handball—and other sports—and, in the process, suffering an occasional injury. If this happens to you, remember that you have help available: a group of homeopathic remedies that can relieve pain, promote healing, and speed you back into the game.

We know many leisure-time athletes who keep these remedies close at hand. Jane, this book's coauthor, whose dream vacation is a ski trip, would almost rather leave her ski boots behind than *Arnica*. Sandy, a public relations person acknowledges that a faulty backhand caused her tennis elbow, but with the help of *Ruta graveolens*, she was soon back on the court improving her swing. John, a young lawyer swears by *Rhus tox.* when he pulls a ligament playing squash.

For a guide to treating your minor sports injuries with a combination of homeopathic remedies and first-aid measures, see the summary quick reference chart at the end of this chapter.

QUICK REFERENCE CHART
REMEDIES FOR BRUISES

Dosage: Two tablets taken 3 or 4 times a day—or, when pain is severe, every 30 minutes to 1 hour. Decrease frequency of dosage as patient improves; discontinue when improvement is well established.

If you are under the care of a homeopathic physician, *do not take any remedies for acute illnesses without checking with your doctor.*

Remedy	General Indications	Worse From	Better From
Arnica	Common bruises Injuries from blow or fall Shock	Least touch Rest	Lying down Head low

Hypericum
(Internally or lotion)
	Crushing injuries to nerves
	Nerve injury to:
	  "Crazybones"
	  Fingertips
	  Nailbeds
	  Palms
	  Soles of feet
	  Tailbones
	  Toes
	Puncture wounds
		Cold
		Touch	

Ledum
(Internally or lotion)
	Bruises:
	  Cold and numb bruised parts
	  Long-lasting
	Black eye, "shiner"
	Splinter under nail
	Bruised nerves
	Puncture wounds
		Warmth	Bathing in cold water

Ruta	Injuries of:
	  Bones
	  Periosteum, bone covering
	  Shins
	  Soft tissue
	Prolapsed, protruding rectum
	Wrist and ankle sprains
		Lying down
		Cold, wet weather	

SPRAINS

Remedy	General Indications	First-Aid Measures
Arnica (Internally or lotion)	Shock of injury Bleeding in tissues	Massage injured area gently with *Arnica* oil or lotion, but only on unbroken skin. Elevate injured part. During the first 24 hours, apply ice bag or cold compress to painful area to reduce swelling and pain; apply heat after that. Wrap injured area with elastic bandage for support.
Bryonia	Injured joint swollen, distended, painful Worse on movement	
Ledum	Injured joint cold and numb Much swelling	
Rhus toxicodendron	After *Arnica* Hot, swollen, painful joint "Rusty gate" feeling; creaky on first movement; better when limbered up	
Ruta graveolens	After *Arnica* Torn and wrenched tendons or ligaments Bruised periosteum (bone covering) Worse in cold wet weather	
Symphytum (Internally and lotion)	After *Arnica* and *Ruta*, if necessary Injury to sinews, tendons, and the bone covering	

Note: If sprain seems severe, seek professional help. Meanwhile, take whichever remedy most closely fits the symptoms.

STRAINS

Remedy	General Indications	First-Aid Measures
Arnica	Sore, bruised feeling Strained back muscles Sore muscles	Elevate the injured part. Apply cold packs during the first 24 hours; heat after that. Wrap loosely with elastic bandage to support injured area.
Rhus toxicodendron	Sore muscles Torn ligaments and tendons Bruised periosteum (bone covering) Worse on first movement, better after limbered up	

Note: If strain seems severe, seek professional help. Meanwhile, take whichever remedy most closely fits the symptoms.

WOUNDS

Remedy	General Indications and Benefits	Worse From	Better From
Arnica	Shock of injury Speeds healing Jagged wounds (internal use only)	Light touch Heat Rest	Head low
Calendula	Cleanses and speeds healing of: 　Abrasions (lotion) 　Scratches (lotion) 　Superficial wounds (lotion)		
Hepar sulphur	Red, swollen, painful wounds	Lying on painful side Slight touch Slightest draft	Warmth
Hypericum	Relieves nerve pain and pain of jagged wounds Cleanses and speeds healing of: 　Jagged, irregular cuts (lotion) 　Lacerations (lotion) 　Painful burns (lotion)	Touch Cold	Bending head backward
Ledum	Cleanses puncture wounds (lotion)	Night Heat of the bed Warm applications	Cold applications

INSECT BITES AND STINGS

Remedy	General Indications	Worse From	Better From
Apis Bee, Hornet, and Wasp Stings	Burning, stinging pains Rapid rosy swelling, not bright red Puffiness rather than hard swelling	Heat Hot applications	
Arnica (Tincture) Bee, Hornet, and Wasp Stings	Applied directly to the sting, relieves pain at once	Least touch Rest	Lying down with head low
Calendula (Tincture) Bee, Hornet, and Wasp Stings	Relieves pain and swelling when applied directly to sting		
Cantharis Bee, Hornet, and Wasp Stings	Red and inflamed stings Burning sensation	Touch Approach	Gentle massage
Carbolicum acidum Poisonous Spider, Scorpion, and Snake Bites	Dusky red face Pale around mouth and nose Listless, sluggish Sensitive to odors		
Crotalus horridus Poisonous Spider, Scorpion, and Snake Bites	Rapid, violent onset of symptoms Much swelling Discoloration around bite	Jarring	
Echinacea Poisonous Spider, Scorpion, and Snake Bites	Red streaks Blood poisoning and infection Sepsis, foul-smelling discharge		
Hypericum (Internally or tincture) Bee, Hornet, and Wasp Stings	Severe pain shooting upward	Cold Touch	Bending head backward
Lachesis Poisonous Spider, Scorpion, and Snake Bites	Affected part dusky red or blue Oozing of dark blood	After sleep	

Note on Bee, Hornet, and Wasp Stings: If victim is allergic to insect stings, rush to nearest hospital emergency room. Meanwhile, give *Apis* in the highest potency you have.

Note on Poisonous Spider, Scorpion, and Snake Bites: Apply an ice pack to the bite to slow the spread of poison, and rush victim to nearest hospital emergency room. Meanwhile, give one of the remedies mentioned here.

INSECT BITES AND STINGS

Remedy	General Indications	Worse From	Better From
Ledum (Internally or tincture) Bee, Hornet, and Wasp Stings	Punctured wounds and stings Numbness or high sensitivity to touch Pains extend upward Wounded parts may be cold	Night Heat of the bed	Cold applications Cold bathing
Oxalicum acidum Poisonous Spider, Scorpion, and Snake Bites	Affected part cold and numb Violent pain Trembling of hands and feet	Slightest touch Thinking about himself	

BURNS

Remedy	Instructions
Arnica	To be given first to prevent shock.
Cantharis	If pain persists after *Arnica*, give 2 tablets every 15 minutes until pain lessens. Repeat *Cantharis* if pain returns.
Causticum	If the pain is accompanied by restlessness and blister formation, give 2 tablets of *Causticum* every 15 minutes until pain lessens.
Aloe Vera Plant	Gel from plant forms a protective covering, relieves pain, and promotes healing.
Calendula Lotion	Immerse burned area in cold water with a few drops of *Calendula* succus or tincture. Saturate dressing with *Calendula* lotion to cleanse, relieve pain, and heal.
OR	
Hypericum Lotion	Immerse burned area in cold *Hypericum* lotion. Dressing should be saturated with *Hypericum* lotion and applied to burned area to prevent serum loss and promote tissue formation.
OR	
Urtica urens Lotion	Soothing lotion when applied externally. Quickly relieves pain and heals. When older burns are characterized by itching and stinging, *Urtica* lotion relieves.

SPORTS INJURIES

Injury	Remedy	First-Aid Measures*
Athlete's Foot	*Calendula*	Wash feet thoroughly with water and mild soap (preferably *Calendula* soap). Apply *Calendula* ointment. Expose feet to air. Avoid synthetic or colored hose.
Bleeding from Mouth	*Calendula*	Rinse mouth with *Calendula* lotion.

Blisters
   Raw burning pains;
   Better from cold applications
	Cantharis	Clean area, bandage to protect from pressure and dirt.

Burning heat	*Urtica*	
Broken Rib Pain	*Bryonia*	Rest in comfortable position. Avoid jarring.
When pain lessens To promote healing of bone	*Symphytum*	
Bruises (Black eye, face bruise, heel or toe bruise, knee bruise, barked skin, strains)	*Arnica*	Cleanse if necessary. Place ice pack over bruise.
Crushed Fingers and Toes	*Hypericum*	Rest and elevate injured part.
Cuts and Abrasions General	*Calendula Lotion*	Clean area gently but thoroughly with mild soap and water, rinse in clear water, then apply *Calendula* lotion. Apply a sterile, nonstick gauze dressing and leave it undisturbed. Keep dressing moistened with *Calendula* lotion.
Nerves (toes, fingers, etc.)	*Hypericum Lotion*	Follow directions above, but substitute *Hypericum* lotion.
Fractures For shock and pain	*Arnica*	Keep patient warm and treat with *Arnica* to prevent shock. Apply ice to painful area. If victim with broken bone must be moved, improvise a splint to keep bones from moving.

*These suggestions are strictly first-aid measures and are not intended to substitute for professional medical treatment. For any serious injury, consult your physician.

SPORTS INJURIES

Injury	Remedy	First-Aid Measures*
Jock Itch	Calendula Lotion or Ointment	Keep groin area clean and dry. Apply Calendula lotion or ointment. Use cornstarch as dusting powder.
Nosebleed		
Profuse bleeding from vigorous nose-blowing	Phosphorus	Sit quietly with head thrown forward. Pinch nostrils together for 5 to 10 minutes.
Bright red blood; gushing	Ipecac	If bleeding continues, pack nostril with plug or sterile gauze. Lie down on your back with head elevated and cold wet cloth across face.
Overexertion Bruised sore feeling Aching muscles and joints General fatigue	Arnica	Rest followed by gentle exercise to limber up muscles. Warm, relaxing bath.
Shin Splints	Arnica	Apply ice pack to reduce pain; then heat treatment and gentle massage.
Sore Muscles	Arnica (Internally and lotion)	Externally, massage injured area with Arnica oil or lotion. Apply cold packs to ease pain; then heat.
Sprained Ankle or Wrist If better from cold applications	Ledum	Massage injured area gently with Arnica oil or lotion, but never on broken skin.
After swelling reduced	Arnica (Internally and lotion)	Elevate the injured part; apply cold pack during first 24 hours; apply heat after that.
After Arnica, if necessary	Ruta graveolens	Support injured joint with loosely wrapped elastic bandage.
If weakness is still present after 2 weeks	Calcarea carbonica	Do as above
Strained Muscles, Tendons, Ligaments	Rhus toxicodendron	Elevate the injured part; apply cold pack during first 24 hours, heat after that Wrap injured area with elastic bandage for support.

*These suggestions are strictly first-aid measures and are not intended to substitute for professional medical treatment. For any serious injury, consult your physician.

SPORTS INJURIES

Injury	Remedy	First-Aid Measures*

Sunstroke and Heat Exhaustion
   Face hot and flushed
   Bursting headache
   Waves of throbbing
	Glonoine	Move victim to cool or shady place.
		Put cold wet cloth on head.
		When conscious give 1 teaspoon of salt in a pint of water; encourage victim to drink several glasses.

Pupils dilated
   Pulse strong, pounding
   Skin burning, dry, flushed
	Belladonna	

Nausea
   Pallor
   Clammy sweat
   Prostration
   Pulse rapid and feeble
	Veratrum album	

Cramping, in addition to *Veratrum album* symptoms	*Cuprum metallicum*	

Tendonitis (Inflamed tendon)
   Painful when beginning to move; better after continued motion
   Worse in damp weather
	Rhus toxicodendron	Wrap with elastic bandage to limit motion in painful joint.

Lame feeling Lacks distinct characteristics of *Rhus tox.*	*Ruta*	
Tennis Elbow	*Ruta*	Apply ice and rest the arm for a few days.
Twisted Knee		Apply cold pack during first 24 hours, heat after that.
Take on first day	*Arnica*	Wrap the injured part to limit motion.
If worse from slightest motion; take on second day	*Bryonia*	Elevate and rest the injured knee.

*These suggestions are strictly first-aid measures and are not intended to substitute for professional medical treatment. For any serious injury, consult your physician.

5

In Case of Emergency

A true emergency is a life-threatening condition. There are only two situations that qualify as *true* emergencies: serious bleeding and obstruction to breathing, both of which will be discussed in this chapter.

Other urgent conditions requiring prompt help such as shock, sudden collapse, poisoning, eye trauma, fever, sunstroke, and heat prostration are usually also considered emergencies, and this chapter will provide you with up-to-date first-aid procedures and a description of one or more indicated homeopathic remedies for these and other situations. For many people, having dental work or surgery seems an emergency, so we have also included remedies to help you before, during, and after undergoing such procedures. Any one of the remedies listed for dental work is appropriate for surgery, so we have grouped them together for your convenience in the end-of-chapter summary table.

Homeopathic remedies both stimulate the body's defense mechanism and make the patient more comfortable. The combination of homeopathy and standard first aid offered in this chapter can make any emergency less of one, even while you are awaiting further medical help.

BLEEDING

To stop bleeding from a cut or injury, press sterile gauze (or the cleanest material available) firmly over the wound. If this doesn't help, apply firm pressure on the blood vessel above the wound. When the bleeding stops, bandage the dressings firmly in place, and take the patient to a doctor.

Choose one of the following internal homeopathic remedies that most closely fits the situation:

Arnica. Your first choice if bleeding has been caused by injury, or if the patient is suffering from shock.

China. Weakness from loss of blood, as indicated by faintness, dimming vision, ringing in ears, and in extreme cases, air hunger (gasping for breath or yawning).

Carbo veg. Where there is steady oozing of dark blood with sudden collapse; cold breath; coldness of limbs; cold, clammy sweat; and air hunger.

Ipecac. Gushes of bright red blood as in a nosebleed, with severe nausea, cold sweat, weak pulse, gasping for breath.

Sabina. When there is threatened abortion and uterine hemorrhage. Remedy may or may not prevent abortion but will improve condition of patient.

Phosphorus. For a profuse nosebleed often caused by vigorous noseblowing, or any type of hemorrhage; when small wounds bleed profusely.

BEYOND FIRST AID: If bleeding has been caused by a pathological condition, a first-aid remedy cannot cure the underlying condition. However, it can help control the bleeding until proper treatment has been given.

OBSTRUCTION TO BREATHING

The brain and other vital organs require a steady supply of life-giving oxygen. Breathing may become obstructed from choking on food or other foreign objects; also, from drowning, allergic swelling of the throat, or severe asthma attack. Prompt action is necessary to restore the flow of oxygen and avoid permanent damage to vital organs.

Choking

The choking victim is unable to speak or breathe. If someone collapses while eating and is not breathing, the person is probably choking. You must act quickly; a person choking on food will usually die in four minutes.

Use one of the two variations of the Heimlich Maneuver, devised by a surgeon, Dr. Henry J. Heimlich, and then administer a remedy if necessary.

Standing Heimlich Maneuver. When the victim is standing or sitting, stand behind him and wrap your arms around the victim's waist. Make a fist with one hand and place it, thumbside in, against the victim's abdomen, slightly above the navel and below the rib cage. Grasp your fist with the other hand, and press into the victim's abdomen with a *quick upward thrust.* Repeat the Heimlich Maneuver several times until food pops out.

Lying-down Heimlich Maneuver. If the victim has collapsed and is too heavy for you to lift, turn the victim face upward and kneel astride the victim's hips. With one hand on top of the other, place the heel of the bottom hand on the abdomen slightly above the navel and below the rib cage. Press into the victim's abdomen with a *quick upward thrust.* Repeat the thrust several times if necessary. If you are a small rescuer who cannot reach around the victim, you can save the person with this position—by using your own body weight to perform the Maneuver.

If the patient suffers from the effects of fright after a choking episode, give a dose of *Aconite. Aconite* is made from the plant monkshood, and was used as a medicine by the ancient Romans. If patient feels bruised and sore as a result of a too-forcefully applied Maneuver, give *Arnica.*

Drowning

Recently, it has been shown that the Heimlich Maneuver can evacuate water from the lungs. Therefore, to revive a drowning victim, first perform the Heimlich Maneuver as for choking. Second, clear the airway as quickly as possible by wiping out the victim's mouth and lowering the head or turning onto the abdomen. Then follow immediately with mouth-to-mouth artificial respiration. If the heart has stopped beating, give complete cardiopulmonary resuscitation, which includes external compression of the chest to massage the heart.

Persist in your efforts until help arrives. Unlike the choking victim, who will die in four minutes unless aided, drowning victims who have been submerged for as long as half an hour have survived.

As soon as possible, give *Antimonium tartaricum*, made from tartrate of antimony. *Antimonium tart.*, one of our valuable remedies from the mineral world, is indicated when the patient is cold and blue, is covered with clammy sweat, has rattling respiration, and is drowning in the body's own secretions, whether from actual drowning or from respiratory or cardiac failure. Dosage: Every ten to fifteen minutes, or until improvement is evident.

Since it is dangerous to put anything in the mouth of an unconscious person, soften two tablets in one-quarter teaspoon of water, and place inside the cheek or under the tongue. The medicine will work as long as it is in contact with the mucous membranes. If the patient is breathing through the mouth and the tissues there are very dry, moisten your finger with a little water before placing the tablets on the inside of the cheek or on the tongue.

Allergic Respiratory Swelling

A rare but serious occurrence is a sudden swelling of the tongue or tissues of the throat, which may close off the airway. This allergic, or anaphylactic, shock may occur after a highly sensitive person has been stung by a bee or has taken penicillin.

Regardless of the type of allergy, *Apis mellifica* has proved lifesaving in this type of respiratory emergency. If you are hypersensitive to bee stings, you would do well to carry *Apis* at all times. If possible, consult a homeopathic physician as to the advisability of carrying high-potency *Apis*.

Asthma Attack

Treatment of asthma is a difficult, complicated medical problem, and should be handled by a physician. While awaiting professional help, you may be able to relieve the symptoms with one of these homeopathic remedies:

Arsenicum album. Patient experiences anxiety and restlessness. Is unable to lie down because of feeling of suffocation that occurs shortly after mid-night.

Carbo vegetabilis. Asthma attack occurs after long, spasmodic coughing spell with gagging and vomiting. Patient feels worse after eating or talking, worse in the evening.

Ipecacuanha. Patient experiences sudden onset of wheezing and feeling of suffocation; coughs constantly but is unable to bring up any mucus. There is a feeling of weight on the chest.

Nux vomica. Asthma attack often follows a stomach upset with much belching. Patient is exceedingly irritable.

SHOCK

Even minor injuries may be accompanied by some degree of shock. You hammer your finger instead of the nail and experience a sudden, clutched feeling in the stomach, increased pulse and breathing rates. The more serious the injury, the greater degree of shock. Symptoms are pale, cold, clammy skin, rapidly rising pulse, restlessness, shallow breathing, a feeling of impending disaster. These symptoms are due to circulatory disturbance and consequent lack of oxygen supply to the nervous system and other tissues.

To lessen shock, reassure the patient. Place on back with legs elevated (except in cases of head or chest injuries, when the head should be slightly higher than the feet). You want the blood to flow to the brain; gravity can help.

Loosen the patient's clothing. Keep patient warm with blankets but avoid overheating as it leads to further loss of fluids by sweating. If person is conscious and thirsty, administer a hot drink such as sweetened tea, but nothing cold.

Arnica is the best remedy for shock. Give *Arnica* every fifteen minutes, then taper off as the patient shows signs of improvement (if necessary, see section on "Drowning" for instructions on giving a remedy to an unconscious person). If the person is agitated, restless, extremely fearful, give *Aconitum napellus* (*Aconite*) instead of *Arnica*.

FAINTING

When for any reason the blood flow to the brain is insufficient to supply needed oxygen, nature forces the person to assume the most favorable position for restoring that supply—the person keels over and lies flat, which helps provide the brain with sufficient oxygen. So note what the wisdom of the body dictates and follow suit. Place the patient face up and loosen tight clothing. Don't allow people to crowd around; this will interfere with the person's air supply.

If the cause of fainting has been determined, one of the following remedies will help:

Chamomilla (German chamomile) From severe pain.

Cinchona officinalis. From loss of blood.

Coffea cruda. From excitement.

Hepar sulphuris (Calcium sulphide). From slight pain.

Pulsatilla nigricans (wind flower). From hot, stuffy atmosphere.

A person who has repeated fainting spells will benefit from constitutional treatment by a homeopathic physician.

BEYOND FIRST AID: A simple faint may be caused by fright, and emotional upset, severe pain, or poor ventilation. On the other hand, a faint may indicate something more serious such as internal bleeding or a heart attack. (A heart attack is usually accompanied by shortness of breath, chest pain, or occasionally, abdominal pain.) If fainting lasts more than a few minutes, keep patient warm and take him or her to a hospital emergency room.

POISONING

Food poisoning is caused by contaminated food or toxic substances such as poisonous berries or mushrooms. The defense mechanism responds to the presence of these dangerous substances, attempting to expel them by vomiting, often accompanied by cramping and weakness.

If the poison is known to be food rather than a corrosive substance or petroleum product, induce the victim to vomit by giving syrup of ipecac, available from drug stores without prescription. Dosage: One tablespoon of syrup of ipecac mixed in one cup of water. (One-half tablespoon for children under one year.) If no vomiting occurs in fifteen minutes, repeat dose. If need be, stick your finger into the victim's throat to induce vomiting.

If this is a case of food poisoning, or ptomaine poisoning, after the vomiting, give *Arsenicum album*. *Arsenicum* is made from deadly poison, arsenic, which, in its homeopathically potentized state, is an effective and safe remedy.

Countless times I've recommended *Arsenicum* for this unpleasant condition, and, thus far, it has never failed me. The other day, Mrs. Jones called in great distress. She knew that the meat she had had in a restaurant the night before had tasted "funny." About 4 A.M., she began vomiting and developed diarrhea. I advised *Arsenicum* every hour, three or four times, then only if vomiting or diarrhea continued or if she felt weak. That day, Mrs. Jones wisely abstained from eating; the next day her appetite returned, and she was back to normal.

Here's where homeopathy works along with your body instead of opposing it. Mrs. Jones's system was trying to get rid of toxic material, an unpleasant but necessary process. The homeopathic remedy gave the defense mechanism a little push in that direction. Taking an antiemetic or antidiarrhea medicine might have forced her body to retain this poisonous matter.

BEYOND FIRST AID: Do not induce vomiting if the poison ingested is a corrosive substance such as acid, ammonia, cleaning fluid, drain cleaner or lye, or a petroleum product such as kerosene, turpentine, or paint thinner. While vomiting, a person could inhale these substances into the lungs, more dangerous than having them in the stomach. Do not induce vomiting if the poison is an unknown substance or if the victim is unconscious. If possible, administer the antidote recommended on the container from which the poison came, or if unknown, dilute the poison in the stomach by giving one teaspoon to one tablespoon of activated charcoal stirred into a glass of water. Repeat frequently. Call your doctor or a poison-control center immediately; keep telephone number of center posted in a prominent place. If you know what the poison was, inform your doctor or take container to the emergency room of your nearest hospital.

EYE INJURIES

In responding to someone's appeal, "I've got something in my eye," do not go digging in the eye; handle it gently, First, try to flush out the speck or foreign body with an eyewash of *Hypericum* lotion (two drops to the eyebath), or plain water. If the person still feels something is there, pull down the lower lid. If you don't see anything, turn back the upper lid by grasping its eyelashes and rolling the lid over a cotton-tipped applicator or pencil. You can safely do this if you can get the patient to relax. If speck is on either lid, try to remove it by touching it lightly with a moistened cotton applicator or moistened corner of a clean handkerchief. Never touch the eye with anything dry.

Aconite, often referred to as "the *Arnica* of the eye," will relieve pain of an eye injury and diminish inflammation, but remember, this effect will be temporary if the foreign body remains.

This was demonstrated to me at a party where one of the women guests was in misery from "something in her eye." It was impossible to examine her eye as she could not open it, so I gave her *Aconite* and offered to take her to a nearby emergency room for treatment. After a few minutes, the eye felt much better, so she decided not to leave the party. The next day I learned that her pain had returned full force an hour after I had left, at which time she sought help at the hospital emergency room, where they removed a sharp-edged chunk of mascara.

BEYOND FIRST AID: If a foreign body in the eye does not come out easily, or if it is on the cornea, cover the eye with a clean cloth and take the person to a physician.

If there is irritation or pain following the removal of a foreign body in the eye, use *Hypericum* or *Calendula* lotion as an eyewash. (One-half teaspoon of tincture to one cup of cool water.)

To control bleeding from a cut eyelid, soak a pad in equal parts of *Calendula* succus and cold water, and apply firm but gentle pressure on the eye. (Succus is a liquid preparation of *Calendula* containing minimal alcohol.)

For a black eye, take *Arnica* internally every hour, if needed, for several hours. If this treatment fails to help and the eye feels better from cold applications, give *Ledum* internally, then apply it in lotion form. If the eye is excessively painful, take *Hypericum* internally.

Many homeopathic physicians believe that *Symphytum officinale* is the best remedy for traumatic injuries of the eye. The ancient Greeks used the medicinal plant for its healing properties. "Symphytum" comes from the Greek "grown together."

In an eye injury, how do we choose among *Arnica*, *Hypericum*, *Ledum*, and *Symphytum*? If there is injury to the eyeball—from a snowball, a tennis ball, or an infant sticking its fist into the mother's eye—give *Symphytum*. If the injury, however, is to the soft tissue of the socket of the eye, as caused by walking into a door or a blow above or below the eye, give *Arnica*. *Ledum* is distinguished by "better from cold," and *Hypericum* is for the injury that is excessively painful.

Although eyestrain is not an emergency situation, you may be interested to know that *Ruta graveolens* can help relieve this condition. This was known to Leonardo and Michelangelo, who brewed tea from rue leaves, which they drank and also used as an eyewash for eyestrain.

FEVER

We have placed "fever" in this chapter on emergencies, but as you learn to understand the workings of the body, you will realize that fever is an ally. Although an elevated temperature does signal a disturbance, the fever is not the disease but a symptom of disease—a useful indicator that the body is engaged in fighting a disease or infection.

Here we again part company with traditional medicine. The ordinary doctor is trained to suppress fever with aspirin or other medications known as febrifuges. The homeopath regards fever as an important part of the healing process. Dr. William Gutman, in his book, *The Little Homeopathic Physician* expresses this concept very well:

> Fever is our strongest weapon in the fight of nature against all bacteria; through its influence all healing reactions are accelerated, the heart beats faster in order to carry the blood, containing all healing matters, quicker to all the organs, respiration is speeded up, thus increasing the intake of the all-important oxygen.

Suppressing fever opposes the healing process, Dr. Gutman writes, "For a real cure, it is necessary to treat with a similar remedy which does not paralyze nature's functions, but supports them."

So, when you develop a fever, we do not treat the fever. We aim to strengthen your body to give it all the help we can to repel the invader. We recommend extra rest, plenty of fluids, a light diet—commonsense measures with which you are probably familiar.

Next, we choose a homeopathic remedy, not based on the fever alone but on the total picture of all your symptoms. This remedy stimulates your body's defense mechanism to deal with the harmful forces. For first-aid purposes, however, certain homeopathic remedies are more frequently indicated in ailments that include fever.

Aconite. Sudden onset of symptoms. Patient is intensely nervous and restless, anxious and fearful. Skin is dry and hot, with a full bounding pulse.

Arsenicum. Patient is fearful and restless and has burning pains relieved by warmth. Very thirsty for frequent sips of water; there is rapid prostration and increasing weakness. Worse after midnight.

Belladonna. Sudden onset of symptoms. Patient has a flushed face, high temperature; pulse is strong and rapid; little or no thirst. May become delirious.

Bryonia. Patient prefers to lie still; worse from the least movement—whether swallowing or turning head or even moving eyes. Very thirsty; drinks large quantities of water. Usually pale and quiet.

Ferrum phosphoricum. Gradual onset of symptoms. Patient has red cheeks and throbbing head as in *Belladonna*, but symptoms are milder. Pulse is fast but not strong; better from cold applications on head.

Gelsemium. Patient is chilly, aches all over, doesn't want to move. Dull headache, droopy eyes, heavy limbs, chills up and down back. Despite fever there is no thirst.

Phosphorus. Patient has fever and chills, night sweats, a thirst for cold drinks. This remedy is often needed when a head cold goes into chest. The sick *Phosphorus* child with a temperature of 104 may appear to be perfectly well. Person may be hungry despite the fever.

Pyrogenium. This is the remedy most often indicated in blood poisoning. Patient's temperature goes up and down, pulse is weak and rapid. Restless, aches all over, has chills, is alternately hot and cold and complains that the bed is hard.

BEYOND FIRST AID: If you develop an unusually high fever, sponging face and forehead with lukewarm water will reduce the fever somewhat and make you more comfortable. If fever persists or continues to rise, contact your physician.

SUNSTROKE

On a hot day, when a person becomes overheated, the cooling mechanism—the evaporation of sweat from the skin—may fail. The victim's skin is hot and dry, body temperature can soar as high as 106 degrees, with the pulse rapid and strong. The person is dizzy, nauseated, weak, and generally has a headache. He or she may vomit, go into convulsions, become delirious.

Choose one of these two homeopathic remedies and give every fifteen to thirty minutes until patient improves.

Belladonna. Victim has burning, dry flushed skin, dilated pupils, a strong pulse.

Glonoine (made from nitroglycerine). Same symptoms as *Belladonna* plus a bursting headache.

Cool the victim off as quickly as possible by pouring liberal amounts of cool water over the skin. Or place a cold compress on the person's head and wrap a cold wet sheet around the body. Give cool drinks to be sipped slowly, but nothing with alcohol or caffeine.

BEYOND FIRST AID: A dry, hot skin, or rapidly rising temperature may indicate a life-threatening emergency. Call an emergency squad. Meanwhile, follow homeopathic and commonsense measures.

HEAT PROSTRATION

This condition is caused by excessive exposure to heat plus dehydration usually attributable to lack of water or to drinking alcoholic beverages. Unlike sunstroke, victim's pulse is not pounding and seldom exceeds 100 beats per minute; the skin is cold and clammy. Other symptoms are similar to those of sunstroke—weakness, dizziness, headache, nausea, blurred vision, irritability, sometimes cramping muscles.

Choose one of these two homeopathic remedies for this condition.

Veratrum album. This remedy is useful in most cases of heat exhaustion. There is prostration with clammy sweat, pallor, nausea, marked weakness, and sometimes rapid pulse.

Cuprum metallicum. If, in addition to *Veratrum alb.* symptoms, the patient suffers from cramps, this is the appropriate remedy.

Have victim rest in a shaded area, or in air-conditioned room, with cold cloths on the head. Urge the person to drink several glasses of water, each with one-half teaspoon of salt.

Prevention, of course, is the best medicine here. In hot weather, drink plenty of fluids and salt your food well, unless advised otherwise by your physician. Abstain from alcoholic drinks if you expect to be out in the sun.

A person who has suffered from either sunstroke or heat prostration is, for some reason, henceforth more susceptible to both these hazards than the average person, and should take extra precautions.

DENTAL WORK

Native Eskimos, before switching to the American diet, had strong, flawless teeth. Few of us are so lucky. Homeopathy cannot prevent tooth decay since heredity and nutrition are major factors, but *Arnica* and other remedies described in this section can take much of the pain and trauma out of dental work.

Melvin G. Henningsen, D.D.S., of Hayward, California, who is well versed in homeopathy, describes *Arnica* as "the dentist's friend, the do-it-all remedy." Dr. Henningsen gives *Arnica* to patients after a dental extraction, scaling (removing debris, calculus, and bacterial plaque from the roots and crowns on the teeth), gum treatment, as well as crown and bridge preparations. *Arnica*, he says, controls pain and bleeding, heals sore gums and tissues, and seems to prevent infection.

Jerome S. Mittelman, D.D.S., of New York City (past president of the International Academy of Preventive Medicine), gives *Arnica* in liquid form to patients: one to two drops for any tissue-traumatizing treatment. "Works wonders," Dr. Mittelman says.

So, if dental surgery is on your agenda, or any extensive dental work, have *Arnica* on hand. Take one dose before and one after your appointment. Take only as often as needed to maintain reasonable comfort.

Recently I had dental surgery to remove the tip of an abscessed root. The oral surgeon told me to take a painkiller before I left the office and to continue treatment round the clock for a few days. He also told me to apply an ice pack during the day and rest, figuring, I suppose, that I'd be prostrated from pain. Being very busy, I ignored all this advice and took *Arnica* instead. I never felt any real discomfort and the incision healed perfectly.

Arnica has been the only remedy I've ever needed as a dental patient, but there are several other remedies to help smooth the dental experience. A business associate was so fearful of going to the dentist that he constantly postponed needed dental work. When a terrible toothache finally drove him to seek help, he was so tense that it was difficult for the dentist to work on him. If this is your problem, consider one of the following remedies before your appointment:

Aconite. If you're excessively nervous and fearful.

Gelsemium. If, in addition to being nervous, you are shaking and have diarrhea.

Chamomilla. If you are hypersensitive to pain; particularly indicated for children.

In addition, if you have had an unpleasant reaction to a dental anesthetic agent, take *Chamomilla* before your appointment. This remedy seems to prevent the "hopped-up" feeling—fast heartbeat, weakness in the legs—that some experience after an anesthetic.

Should you be in pain after your appointment, there are several remedies to relieve different types of discomfort. If there is nerve pain—a sharp, electric pain—from drilling, take *Hypericum*. If there is deep aching, as when the periosteum (the thin layer between gum and bone) has been injured, take *Ruta*. In addition, *Ruta* will often help a condition called "dry socket." This occurs after extractions when too vigorous rinsing dislodges the blood clot that protects the newly exposed nerve from air. Obviously, one should avoid rinsing too energetically.

There are remedies to help you in other dental situations. *Chamomilla* heals a painful needle wound resulting from an injection. If the puncture wound feels cold, *Ledum* is the best choice. *Phosphorus* will control excessive, stubborn bleeding.

Calendula lotion is effective as a mouthwash to promote healing of the mouth after deep scaling, or any painful dental treatment. If you have denture or canker sores, saturate a cotton applicator with the lotion and apply it to the spot. To prepare *Calendula* lotion, add one-half teaspoon of *Calendula* succus to a cup of water.

SURGERY

Arnica, which controls shock and soreness, heals bruised tissues and controls bleeding, is an indispensable remedy to take before and after surgery. Margerie B. Blackie, in her book, *The Patient, Not the Cure*, recalls a surgeon who knew the value of *Arnica*. "Whenever I attended an operation upon one of my patients, he used to greet me with, 'Blackie, have you given *Arnica*?"

I tell all my patients who are undergoing surgery to take *Arnica*. Dosage: two tablets of *Arnica* before and after surgery; repeat as often as needed.

The other day, a patient, Kay, told me that her teenage daughter had recently had an appendectomy. "I put a crushed tablet of *Arnica* under her tongue as soon as she was even conscious," Kay said. (Or, you can soften two tablets in a quarter-teaspoon of water.) Kay also related how impressed the surgeon was with her daughter's recovery. "He showed off her incision to all the nurses!"

In addition, if a patient is unusually anxious and apprehensive before surgery, I suggest taking *Aconite* the night before the operation and the next day. *Gelsemium*, taken preoperatively, will also calm the patient who is practically trembling with fear.

Some patients find it difficult to recover from any general anesthetic; they have prolonged postoperative vomiting and come out of the anesthetic slowly. One dose of *Phosphorus* taken the night before the operation seems to alleviate this reaction to anesthesia.

QUICK REFERENCE CHART

REMEDIES FOR EMERGENCIES

Dosage: Two tablets, taken 3 or 4 times a day or, when pain is severe, every 30 minutes to 1 hour. Decrease frequency of dosage as patient improves; discontinue when improvement is well established.

If you are under the care of a homeopathic physician, *do not take any remedy for acute ailments without checking with your doctor.*

Remedy	General Indications	Worse From	Better From
Aconite For Eye Injury	To diminish inflammation To relieve pain	Night Warm room	Open air
For Conditions with fever	Sudden onset Restless Fearful	Lying on painful side	
Apis mellifica For Breathing difficulty	Allergic shock Reactions to bee stings Throat passages closed Tongue swollen	Heat Hot applications Touch Pressure	Motion Cold bath Open air
Antimonium tartaricum For Breathing difficulty	Cardiac failure: drowning in own secretions Drowning: cold and blue patient; respiration rattling Respiratory failures: drowning in own secretion; clammy sweat	Evening Lying down at night Warmth	Sitting erect Belching Expectoration
Arnica For Bleeding	Caused by injury	Least touch	Lying down
For Eye injury	Black eye Injury to socket, soft tissue surrounding eye	Rest	Head low
For Shock	From injury		
Arsenicum album For Asthma	Unable to lie down, afraid of suffocation Wheezing respiration Great debility Burning in chest Worse from 1 to 2 A.M.	After midnight Cold	Warmth Head elevated Warm drinks
For Conditions with fever	Restless Anxious Burning pains Thirsty for frequent small sips		
For Food poisoning	Vomiting and diarrhea		

EMERGENCIES

Remedy	General Indications	Worse From	Better From
Belladonna For Conditions with fever	Sudden onset Violent symptoms Face flushed Skin burning to the touch Restless	Afternoon Lying down Touch Jarring Noise	Being semierect
For Sunstroke	Pupils dilated Pulse strong, pounding Skin burning, dry, flushed		
Bryonia For Conditions with fever	Thirsty for large drinks Skin pale Irritable Desires quiet	Motion Touch Warmth	Rest Quiet
Calendula (lotion) For Eye injury	Control of bleeding		

Carbo vegetabilis
For Asthma
	Onset after long spasmodic
	  coughing spell with gagging
	  and vomiting
	Sore, raw chest with difficult
	  breathing, especially in evening
	Air hunger; must be fanned
	Bluish face; cold breath
	Symptoms worse after eating or
	  talking
		Evening
		Open air
		Warm, damp
		  weather
		Wine
			Belching
			Fanning

For Bleeding, External or Internal	Dark blood, steady oozing		
For Collapse	From any cause Air hunger Cold breath Sweat, cold and clammy		
Chamomilla For Fainting	From severe pain	Night Open air	Being carried Warm wet weather
For Intolerance of pain		Heat Anger	
China For blood loss resulting in:	Air hunger (gasping for breath) Faintness Ringing in ears Dimming of vision	Slightest touch Draft After eating Loss of vital fluids	Hard pressure Open air. Warmth
For Aftereffects of loss of any vital fluids	With weakness and any of the above		
Coffea For Fainting	From excitement	Excessive emotions Strong odors	Warmth Lying down
For Sleeplessness	From excitement or joy	Noise Open air Cold	Holding ice in mouth

EMERGENCIES

Remedy	General Indications	Worse From	Better From
Cuprum metallicum For Heat exhaustion	Cramping in addition to *Veratrum album* symptoms	Contact Vomiting	Perspiring Drinking cold water
Ferrum phosphoricum For Conditions with fever	Red cheeks Gradual onset Soft and rapid pulse	Right side Night 4 to 6 A.M. Touch Jar Motion	Cold applications
Gelsemium For Conditions with fever	Aching Chilly Drooping eyes	10 A.M. Excitement Damp weather	Open air Continued motion Profuse urination
For Influenza	Lethargic		
Glonoine For Sunstroke	Face hot and flushed Bursting headache Waves of throbbing Skin sweaty	Left side 6 A.M. to noon Motion Jarring Stooping Lying down	Brandy
Hepar sulphur For Fainting	From slight pain	Dry, cold weather	Warmth After eating Damp weather
Hypericum For Eye injury	Excessive and long-lasting pain Pain after removal of foreign object (lotion as an eyewash)	Cold Touch	Bending head backward
Ipecacuanha For Asthma	Sudden onset Wheezing; gasps for air Must sit up to breathe Violent, rattling cough with every breath Unable to bring up any mucus Suffocates and gags with cough Feeling of weight on chest	Time to time Moist, warm wind Lying down	
For Bleeding	Bright red blood, gushing Gasping for air Nosebleed Severe nausea Weak pulse Cold sweat		
Ledum For Eye injury (internally and lotion)	For pain after *Arnica* fails to relieve	Night Heat of the bed	Cold applications

EMERGENCIES

Remedy	General Indications	Worse From	Better From
Nux vomica For Asthma	Attack often follows stomach upset with much belching Oppressed breathing with shallow respiration Tight, dry, hacking cough Cough brings on bursting headache Irritable Hypersensitive	Morning Mental exertion After eating Dry weather Cold Touch	Evening Uninterrupted nap Damp wet weather Strong pressure
Phosphorus For Bleeding	Profuse bleeding anywhere Nosebleed: profuse or from vigorous blowing	Twilight Lying on left or painful side	Lying on right side Dark Cold
For Conditions with fever	Thirst for cold drinks Appears well despite high temperature Colds travel to chest Cough Sweats at night	Touch Physical or mental exertion Warm food or drink Getting wet in hot weather Ascending stairs	Cold food Open air Sleep Washing in cold water
Pulsatilla For Fainting	From hot, stuffy atmosphere	Heat After eating	Open air Motion Cold applications
Pyrogen For Conditions with fever	Aching Pulse and temperature out of proportion Restless; bed feels too hard		Motion
For Blood poisoning			
Ruta graveolens For Eye injury	Eye-strain followed by headache Painful, red, hot eyes	Lying down Cold, wet weather	
Sabina For Bleeding	Uterine hemorrhage	Least motion Heat Warm air	Cool fresh air
Symphytum For Eye injury	Injury to eyeball Pain in eye following a blow of blunt object		
Veratrum album For Heat exhaustion	Nausea Pallor Prostration Pulse rapid and feeble Clammy sweat Weakness	Night Wet, cold weather	Walking Warmth

DENTAL PROBLEMS AND SURGERY

Remedy	Specific Indications	General Indications
Aconite		
For Dental problems	Fear of treatment	Anxiety
		Fear
For Surgery	Fear of surgery	Nervousness
Arnica	Sore gums	
For Dental problems	Soreness after tooth extraction	Bleeding
		Pain
For Surgery	Soreness following surgery	Bruised tissue
		Injury to soft tissue
		Infection
		To promote healing
		Shock
Calendula lotion (½ tsp. *Calendula* succus to 1 cup water)	Canker sores	Infection
	Dental sores	To promote healing
	Promote healing after deep scaling	Pain
For Dental problems (as a mouthwash)	Pain following treatment	
For Surgery	Promote healing of surgical wound	
	Pain following surgery	
Chamomilla		
For Dental problems	Needle wound from injections	Hypersensitivity to pain, especially in children
Gelsemium		
For Dental problems	Apprehensive about treatment	Loose bowels from fright, excitement
For Surgery	Trembling, fearful preoperative patient	Fear
		Shaking
Hypericum	Nerve pain from drilling	
For Dental problems	Root canal discomfort	Injuries to nerves
	Tooth extraction	
Ledum	Puncture wound from injection	Wound cold
For Dental problems		Wound relieved by cold applications
Phosphorus		
For Dental problems	Excessive bleeding	Profuse bleeding anywhere
Ruta	Deep aching	"Bruised" bones; bone covering injured
For Dental problems	"Dry socket"	

6
How to Prevent and Treat Colds, Coughs, and Earaches

COLDS, coughs, and earaches frequently occur at the same time. The "common cold" is an upper respiratory viral infection that affects nasal passages and throat. A cough is an attempt to clear the air passages of irritating mucus. Since the lining of the throat is continuous with that of the eustachian tube to the ear, swelling and discomfort often extend from the throat into the ears.

Homeopathy can help all of these conditions, including flu (influenza), a viral infection that is more severe than a cold. Looking through the group of remedies listed in each section, you may wonder at the duplication. For example, *Belladonna* and *Pulsatilla* are indicated for colds, coughs, and earaches. This is so because these conditions present so many of the same symptoms, and, as you already know, a remedy is prescribed on the basis of symptoms rather than on the so-called disease. Whether the problem is bacterial infection or congestion of the throat or earache, the medicine that most closely matches your symptoms will shorten the course of the ailment and prevent any serious consequences.

COLDS

Homeopathy offers no single remedy for "colds." But we have a choice of safe and effective remedies for the vast number of people who get colds. To select the right one, you must carefully observe symptoms and spend a little time learning the characteristics of each remedy. Armed with this knowledge, you will be able to select a remedy that not only relieves symptoms but also promotes early recovery from that cold.

The following homeopathic remedies are indicated for colds. Make your selection carefully. Although homeopathic medicines are safe and nontoxic, too many remedies in succession are like contradictory orders from a control tower to a pilot; they confuse the defense mechanism.

Aconite. To be taken at the first sign of a cold after exposure to dry, cold wind. Useful only during the onset of a cold. Symptoms are frequent sneezing, burning throat, thirst, and restlessness at night.

Allium cepa. Sneezing accompanied by streaming eyes and nose. Nasal discharge makes the nose and upper lip sore. Patient feels better in open air. Coughing hurts the larynx.

Antimonium tartaricum. You can hear the rattling of mucus in the chest. The patient, if a child or an elderly person, has difficulty spitting up mucus. Is weak and drowsy, with a sweaty, pale face; often gasps for breath. Feels better upon sitting up, worse on lying down and worse in the evening.

Arsenicum. A thin, watery nasal discharge irritates the nostrils and upper lip. The keynote is burning pains that are relieved by heat. The throat is relieved by hot drinks. Patient feels better indoors even though nose is stopped up. Head colds tend to go down into the chest. There may be dry cough; everything feels worse after midnight.

Belladonna. At the sudden onset of cold, patient has a flushed face, skin that feels hot and dry to the touch. Fever often strikes quickly, along with restlessness and sensitivity to light. The sore throat is often bright red, worse on the right side. Patient may suffer from a short, dry, tickling cough that is worse at night. Infrequent thirst is another symptom.

Bryonia. The *Bryonia* patient is often known as "the bear," wanting to be left alone and lying perfectly still, growling when disturbed. Symptoms are worse with the slightest movement. Is thirsty for large amounts of cold drinks. The cold tends to travel into the chest. The cough is hard and dry, often accompanied by chest pains and a bursting headache, and is aggravated if patient steps into a warm room. Lips and mouth are dry, but the patient may have watery discharge and a stuffy nose.

Dulcamara. This is the reverse of *Gelsemium*, the cold coming on when the weather or temperature suddenly changes from hot to cold. There is a profuse watery discharge from nose and eyes, and the nose runs more in a warm room than a cold one.

Euphrasia. Contrary to *Allium cepa*, a profuse watery nasal discharge from the nose and eyes makes the eyes but not the nose sore. The discharge is worse at night, when the patient is lying down. Conversely, the cough is worse by day, but better when the patient is lying down.

Ferrum phos. When a beginning cold is accompanied by a slight fever, *Ferrum phos.* is often indicated. This remedy has proved useful in the early stages of many infections, but it is difficult to find any firm guidelines for its use as it did not bring out distinctive symptoms in proving.

Gelsemium. Warm, moist weather often brings on the slow onset of this cold. The patient feels sluggish, chilly, and has a dull headache with a heavy feeling in the eyes and limbs. Wants to be left alone. There is much sneezing and a watery discharge that irritates the nose, but there is seldom any thirst.

Hepar sulphuris. The cold is apt to develop in cold, dry weather, with a sticking sensation in back of throat that feels like a splinter. The cold spreads from throat to ear. Pain extends to the ears on swallowing. Nasal discharge is yellow. The cough has a rattling sound and the patient may cough up thick yellow mucus. Extremely sensitive to drafts, the patient is both chilly and sweaty, with perspiration that smells sour.

Mercurius. For a cold that begins with creeping chilliness. There is much sneezing, with raw smarting nostrils. Either a thick yellow-green nasal discharge or a profuse watery discharge irritates the nose and upper lip. Saliva accumulates because it hurts to swallow. A bad odor emanates from the mouth and the whole person smells sick.

Natrum muriaticum. Begins with sneezing and a nasal discharge that is either watery or of the consistency of egg white, and irritates the nose. The nose becomes stopped up and there is a loss of smell and taste. A cough may develop, with stitches in chest. Often patient has a bursting headache and fever blisters. Is annoyed by sympathy.

Nux vomica. During the early stages of a cold. Person has sneezing spells; nose runny during the daytime and stopped up at night. Throat is sore and person is irritable. Feels chilly at the slightest movement, is worse when exposed to cold air, and may develop a painful cough.

Pulsatilla (from wind flowers). For "ripe" cold with thick, creamy yellow discharge. The nose is stuffed up at night and indoors, flows in open air. Despite a fever, the patient is not thirsty. Is apt to be weepy and wants attention and sympathy. Craves open air; better from moving about. The lips are chapped, and peel.

If a headache accompanies your cold, consult the section on headaches, in chapter 10 on women. We have placed this subject here because women are more prone to headaches, but this material is also relevant to men.

Linus Pauling believes that large doses of vitamin C are effective in averting a cold. Other researchers disagree. We don't know the answer. Patients repeatedly tell us that they have aborted colds and other respiratory infections by taking high doses of vitamin C. Therefore, I suggest that you take 500 to 1000 milligrams of ascorbic acid (vitamin C) every hour or two. If bowels become loose or burning, this may indicate that you are excreting excess ascorbic acid; cut back and symptoms will subside.

Vitamin A seems to be beneficial for tissue covering and lining the nose and throat as well as the urinary and intestinal tracts. Take at least 20,000 or 25,000 units per day.

To prevent future colds, consider one of the precepts of holistic health: Illness is a signal that some aspect of your life deserves attention and reform. As Edward Bauman, editor of *The Holistic Health Handbook*, expresses it: "We need to allow ourselves the opportunity to rest, reflect, and rejuvenate—and to come to terms with the behavior that was originally responsible for our disease." You might also consider whether this cold may be a handy escape hatch. A young friend repeatedly caught cold until she figured out that this usually occurred when she wanted to avoid an obligation or when she felt stressed. Even though you may recall a specific occasion on which you were exposed to the highly contagious cold virus, the question remains: why were you susceptible at that particular time?

BEYOND FIRST AID: A cold isn't always a viral infection. Watery nose and eyes may be an allergic reaction, or due to sinus congestion. A sore throat may be the beginning of a serious illness. If symptoms persist, consult your physician.

For the Pain and Discomfort of a Cold...

Aspirin manufacturers have led us to believe that aspirin is good for a cold. These claims, according to a report submitted to the Food and Drug Administration of America in 1977, are "subtly misleading if not downright deceptive." Aspirin is *not* safe for everybody and *not* harmless (see chapter 10).

Heavily advertised cold and cough remedies contain, in addition to aspirin, an antihistamine to dry up nasal secretions. This ingredient, according to Dr. Sol Katz, head of the pulmonary disease division at Georgetown University Hospital, is "worthless, expensive, and harmful." A leading allergist, Ben Feingold, M.D., states that "antihistamine drugs neither prevent nor cure the 'common cold' .... Antihistamines may in some cases influence the severity of the symptoms of the 'common cold,' but the cause remains unaffected, and the course of the illness is not shortened."

FLU

Influenza, commonly called flu, manifests symptoms of chills and fever, headache, general aches and pains. In uncomplicated cases, the acute symptoms usually last for only a few days.

If you come down with flu, consider the following remedies:

Arsenicum album. Patient is restless, fearful, aching, and irritable. Is thirsty for sips of water and is better from warm drinks, worse from cold ones. Dislikes the smell, or even the sight, of food. Has burning pains here and there, and usually feels worse after midnight.

Bryonia. Patient has a painful cough and pain in the throat and chest. Everything feels worse from even the slightest motion. Patient is irritable, quiet, wants to be left alone. Is usually very thirsty, with dry mouth and lips.

Eupatorium perfoliatum. Patient experiences a deep aching in the bones and even the eyeballs are sore. May feel totally "wiped out," unable to exert the least effort. Is usually thirsty, especially as the chill begins to come on.

Gelsemium. There is gradual onset of chilling, aching, lassitude, and fever. Patient is not thirsty. Persistently apathetic and indifferent to life. Lies quietly, eyelids drooping.

Nux vomica. Nux vomica is sometimes indicated when a cold has developed into influenza. The patient is irritable, chilly, sensitive to noises and odors, worse from cold or open air. Is better lying down and from warmth.

Phosphorus. Often the patient doesn't show the severity of the illness. A child, for example, with a temperature of 104 degrees may play happily. Colds that go down into the chest, accompanied by a dry, tight cough, often respond to *Phosphorus.* Patient may feel very weak. Is thirsty for refreshing ice-cold drinks, but may vomit as soon as the water is warm in the stomach. Has laryngitis with or without pain, and may lose voice completely.

Many people all over the world have avoided flu by taking the homeopathic "cold and flu" tablet. Dosage: one tablet every two to four weeks throughout the flu season. This tablet is made from the combined strains of influenza virus from the major flu epidemics since 1918. The combined strains are then homeopathically prepared and potentized. No ill effects have ever been reported from the "cold and flu" tablet, and the rate of protection has been high. In the flu epidemic of 1918 to 1920, the homeopaths lost only 1 per cent of their patients, as opposed to 30 to 40 per cent under allopathic care. Fortunately, allopathic treatment today is more effective than in the twenties.

As antibiotics do not affect viral diseases such as influenza, ordinary medicine has very little to offer in the treatment of flu.

BEYOND FIRST AID: The influenza virus weakens the body's defenses against bacteria, and there is the risk of developing a secondary pneumonia. Therefore, the person recovering from an attack of influenza must be very careful not to get chilled or overtired. If symptoms worsen or linger, see your doctor.

COUGHS

Coughing is an effective way of keeping foreign matter out of the delicate air passages. The presence of an irritant such as bacteria, dust, or pollen in the lower parts of the respiratory system stimulates the production of mucus, which coats and flushes out the undesirable material. Such a cough will sound "juicy," telling you that there is something down there to be coughed up. Do not suppress your cough with any form of cough medicine. By doing so, you are blocking the protective mechanism of the body that is trying to expel the mucus to prevent a deeper infection.

For remedies to help a cough, consider these remedies that have cough symptoms.

Aconite. The cough comes on suddenly after exposure to cold dry wind. A constant short, dry cough with a croupy sound wakens the patient from sleep. Awakens with a sense of anxiety. Cough arises from the larynx when patient enters a warm room.

Belladonna. Person is red-faced, burning hot, with dilated pupils. The cough begins as if a speck had settled in larynx. Sudden onset; dry, teasing cough keeps household awake at night.

Bryonia. A hard, dry cough hurts the chest and necessitates sitting up in bed. As with *Aconite,* the cough becomes worse when entering a warm room. Worse from movement: patient is thirsty for cold drinks; irritable, wanting to be left alone.

Ferrum Phos. A short, painful cough from irritation or tickling in the windpipe.

Hepar sulph. This is another remedy indicated by oversensitivity, especially to cold air and the slightest draft. Patient wants to be wrapped up and can't bear to be uncovered; even putting a hand out of bed may start a coughing spell. Cough is loose, rattling, and croupy; patient may cough up thick yellow mucus. Sometimes a coughing spell causes strangling and gagging.

Kali bichromicum. The cough has a brassy and hacking sound that seems to come from a tickle at the base of the throat. Expectoration is long strings of ropy, tough mucus that may be yellowish.

Nux vomica. A dry, teasing cough; sore larynx and chest. Cough may come in spells and end with retching; more apt to occur in cold, dry, windy weather. Patient often feverish; shivers when moving or uncovered. Oversensitive to noise, odors, light, or music; easily offended.

Phosphorus. This remedy is often indicated when a head cold has gone into the chest. A dry, tickling, exhausting cough may come from the larynx or farther down in the chest. Patient may feel sensation of tightness across the chest or as if a great weight were pressing on it. Cough is induced by talking or by being in the open air. May have a bursting headache. Thirsty for ice-cold drinks and fruit juices.

Pulsatilla. There is a dry cough in the evening but it sounds loose in the morning. Patient may have paroxysms of coughing with gagging and choking, and will bring up thick yellowish mucus. The cough is worse on coming into a warm room and, as always with *Pulsatilla* the person is better in the open air. May feel as if there is a weight on the chest.

Rumex crispus. (made from a plant known as yellow dock). One of its symptoms is the opposite of *Aconite*: cough occurs when going outside. Person has dry, short paroxysms of coughing or a constant hack.

Spongia. Patient wakens from sleep with a suffocating feeling; difficulty in breathing. Anxious as with croup. A loud cough sounding like sawing through a board; worse from talking.

As any concert or theatergoer knows, cough can be dry or rattling, or start with a tickle high in the throat. For immediate relief, suck a slippery elm lozenge, black currant pastille or lemon drop. Or, if you're at home, make your own cough mixture of equal parts honey, glycerine, and lemon juice; take a half-teaspoon and hold in the mouth as long as possible. Avoid all medicated cough drops; they contain camphor, menthol, eucalyptus or chloroform, all of which render a homeopathic remedy useless.

If cough remedies temporarily make you feel better, there's a reason: most are loaded with alcohol. Vick's contains 25 percent alcohol. It's not the alcohol that's so harmful; it's the action of the medicine, which suppresses the cough. As Dr. Ben Feingold explains it: "Suppression of the cough prevents natural elimination of bronchial secretions."

EARACHES

Occasionally, a common cold may extend into the ears. Warmth from a hot water bottle or propping up the head may relieve the pain.

The following homeopathic remedies have brought relief to persons suffering from earache:

Aconite. Sudden earache after a chill and exposure to cold. Ear is red hot and painful and better from warm applications.

Belladonna. Sudden onset, particularly when the right ear is affected. Patient has a dry, flushed face: dry, burning skin; is restless and thirstless.

Chamomilla. Patient is oversensitive and intolerant of pain, which makes for extreme irritability and even rudeness. The person needing *Chamomilla* is never calm. Sometimes one cheek is red and hot, the other pale and cold. Pain is worse from warm applications.

Ferrum phos. This is the most commonly indicated remedy for the early stages of an earache. The proving symptoms are not very distinctive, but the remedy has proved to be very helpful in the beginning stage of an inflammation such as occurs in an ear infection.

Hepar sulph. Person is worse from any draft, and wants to be well covered. Is irritable, complains of stitching pains, and is sensitive to touch.

Kali muriaticum (potassium chloride). Earache and diminished hearing, with cracking noises on blowing the nose and swallowing. Person has a stuffy sensation in the ear and the ear feels closed. *Kali mur.* is also indicated when the patient's hearing is impaired after the earache has subsided.

Magnesia phosphorica. This is a nerve remedy. Earache in this remedy is usually from exposure to cold wind rather than an infection. The right ear is most often affected. Pain is worse from washing face and neck in cold water. The strongest characteristic is relief from warmth.

Mercurius. Earache in damp or changeable weather, worse at night. Patient is sweaty and smells sick. A large, flabby tongue shows imprint of teeth on the edges; there is much saliva and bad breath.

Pulsatilla. Redness and swelling in the external ear. Person experiences severe throbbing pains and ears feel as if they are stopped up. Worse from warmth and from becoming overheated, worse in the evening and at night. Patient craves fresh air and is often weepy.

BEYOND FIRST AID: Although a rare occurrence in an adult, an earache may be a warning of a middle-ear infection. Occasionally, the external ear becomes inflamed and painful. If you experience such symptoms, see your doctor.

QUICK REFERENCE CHART
REMEDIES FOR COLDS, COUGHS, AND EARACHES

Dosage: Two tablets taken 3 or 5 times a day or, when pain is severe, every 30 minutes to 1 hour. Decrease frequency of dosage as patient improves; discontinue when improvement is well established.

If you are under the care of a homeopathic physician, *do not take any remedies for acute illnesses without checking with your doctor.*

Remedy	Specific Indications	Guiding Symptoms	Worse From	Better From
Aconite For Colds	First stages of common cold Frequent sneezing Dripping of clear, hot fluid from nose, especially in morning Burning throat, sensitive to touch Throbbing, congestive headache Roaring in ears	Onset after exposure to cold, dry wind Sudden onset Frightened Restless at night Thirsty Fever One cheek red, the other pale	Evening and night Warm room Lying on affected side Music Tobacco smoke Dry, cold winds	Open air
For Coughs	First remedy for croup Patient wakens anxiously with croupy-sounding cough Constant short, dry cough Cough begins when coming into warm room			
For Earache	External ear red, hot, painful, swollen Warm applications relieve pain Sensation as if drop of water in left ear			
Allium cepa For Colds	Sneezing Streaming eyes and nose Constant watery discharge, sometimes from only one nostril Burning nasal discharge makes nose and upper lip sore Inflammation soon spreads to ears Tickling cough causing tearing pain in throat; patient grasps throat Rawness in throat, extending down into chest	Headache, mostly in forehead Hoarseness, beginning laryngitis Symptoms begin on left side and extend toward right	Evening Warm room	Open air Cold room

COLDS, COUGHS, AND EARACHES

Remedy	Specific Indications	Guiding Symptoms	Worse From	Better From
Antimonium tartaricum For Colds	Rattling of mucus in chest Difficulty spitting up mucus, especially in elderly people and children	Weak Drowsy Sweaty, pale face Feels cold Gasps for breath	Evening Lying down Warmth Damp, cold weather Sour foods or liquids Milk	Sitting up Cold, open room Expectoration
Arsenicum For Colds	Profuse, thin, watery nasal discharge irritating nose and upper lip Red eyes and nose Much sneezing Head colds tend to go down into chest Sore throat relieved by hot drinks	Chilly Burning pains relieved by heat Restless Anxious Weak and exhausted Thirsty for small, frequent sips	Lying on right side After midnight Sight or smell of food Cold drinks	Elevating head Hot drinks Hot applications
For Influenza	Aching Aversion to sight and smell of food Tendency to diarrhea and vomiting, especially after eating or drinking			
Belladonna For Colds	Bright-red sore throat, sometimes worse on right side	Sudden and violent onset Skin red, dry, hot to touch Flushed face Burning fever Restless Eyes sensitive to light, pupils dilated Thirstless	Lying down Motion Jarring Noise Light	Standing Sitting erect
For Coughs	Short, dry, frequent cough, worse at night Cough begins as if speck had gotten in throat Tickling and burning in throat with violent coughing spasms			
For Earache	Sudden onset, especially when earache is in right ear Tearing pain in middle and external ear Throbbing pain deep in ear, tempo of heartbeat Child cries out in sleep from pain			

COLDS, COUGHS, AND EARACHES

Remedy	Specific Indications	Guiding Symptoms	Worse From	Better From
Bryonia For Colds	Head cold travels to chest Hard, dry, racking cough with painful chest Watery nasal discharge with stuffy nose	Wants to be left alone Wants to lie perfectly still Irritable Thirsty for large amounts of cold drinks	Light touch Eating or drinking Slightest motion Warm room Warmth	Firm pressure Rest Cold Lying on affected side because it prevents motion
For Coughs	Hard, dry, racking cough causing pain in chest, stomach Presses hand to chest when coughing Coughing causes bursting headache Worse at night, causes patient to sit up in bed	Lips and mouth dry Urine dark and scanty		
For Influenza	With painful cough Painful throat and chest			
Chamomilla For Earache	Soreness and severe pain Stitching pains Ears feel stopped Frantic from pain	Intolerant of pain Extremely irritable Sensitive One cheek red, the other pale Thirsty	Night Warm applications Heat Open air, wind	Being carried Warm, wet weather
Dulcamara For Colds	Profuse watery discharge from nose and eyes Cold air and cold rain cause nose to stop up Eyes red and sore Sore throat	Onset after cold, wet weather Onset after getting wet, or chilled when heated	Night Cold Rainy weather	Moving about External warmth
Eupatorium For Influenza	Deep aching in back and limbs, as if bones were broken Bursting headache Afraid to move because of pain Eyeballs sore Insatiable thirst followed by chills and fever Vomiting preceded by thirst May be vomiting of bile	Great weakness Soreness	Time to time Tight clothing	Conversation

COLDS, COUGHS, AND EARACHES

Remedy	Specific Indications	Guiding Symptoms	Worse From	Better From
Euphrasia For Colds	Profuse bland nasal discharge Streaming eyes, sore from discharge Discharge worse at night and when lying down Hawking up of offensive mucus Hard cough worse by day and when lying down		Indoors Warmth Light	Open air Dark Coffee
Ferrum phosphoricum For Colds	Beginning stages Red, burning eyes	Beginning stages of all inflammatory problems	Right side Touch Motion Jarring	Cold applications
For Coughs	Early stages Short, painful, tickling cough, better at night Hard, dry cough with sore chest Bronchitis First stages, before ear abscesses Throbbing pain	Gradual onset of fever Pale complexion with red cheeks Soft, rapid pulse Hoarseness Restlessness Sleeplessness		
Gelsemium For colds	Summer colds Much sneezing Watery nasal discharge that irritates nose Feels as if hot water is dripping from nostrils Dry cough	Drowsy, sluggish Chilly Tiredness and aching of whole body Drooping eyelids Headache as if band around head	Damp weather Tobacco smoking Anticipation, even of pleasurable events Thinking about ailments	Continued motion Bending forward Profuse urination Open air
For Influenza	Tiredness of whole body Head, eyelids, limbs feel heavy Fever, but no thirst Cold with chills up and down back	Scalp sore to touch Mild fever Lack of thirst Wants to be left alone Apathy, indifference to life Symptoms develop several days after exposure to warm, moist weather		

COLDS, COUGHS, AND EARACHES

Remedy	Specific Indications	Guiding Symptoms	Worse From	Better From
Hepar sulphur For Colds	Cold begins with irritation in throat Nasal discharge, first watery then thick and yellow Infection spreads from throat to ear Splinter sensation in back of throat	Onset after exposure to cold, dry weather Extremely sensitive to drafts Chilly Hoarse Sweating, with sour odor Peevish	Lying on painful side Cool air Slightest draft Touch	Warmth Wrapping head up After eating
For Coughs	Dry, hoarse cough Loose, rattling croupy cough, worse in morning Cough when any part of body gets cold or uncovered, or when eating anything cold May cough up thick yellow mucus			
For Earache	Sticking pains from throat to ears on swallowing Wants to be wrapped up; ears covered			
Kali bichromicum For Cough	Cough with brassy sound Brings up tough, stringy mucus	Voice hoarse, worse in evening Thick, stringy discharges	Morning Hot weather Undressing	Lying down Heat
Kali muriaticum Ear Earache	Snapping and noise in the ear Impaired hearing following earache To clear eustachian tube following earache		Motion Rich foods Fats	
Magnesia phosphorica For Earache	Without respiratory infection "Nerve" pain—sharp, aching, jerking or tearing Intermittent pain, not steady	Onset after exposure to cold wind Tired and exhausted	Right side Night Cold Cold air Touch	Warmth Pressure Rubbing

COLDS, COUGHS, AND EARACHES

Remedy	Specific Indications	Guiding Symptoms	Worse From	Better From
Mercurius For Colds	Begins with creeping chilliness Much sneezing Thick green nasal discharge or profuse watery discharge Discharge makes nose and upper lip sore Smarting raw sore throat Difficult swallowing	Profuse salivation Coated tongue with bad odor from mouth Person smells sick No relief from sweating Very thirsty, even though mouth is moist Weak and trembling	Night Lying on right side Wet, damp weather Perspiration Warm room Warm bed	
For Earache	Abscessed ears Sticking pains, worse at night			
Natrum muriaticum For Colds	Begins with sneezing Nasal discharge watery or like egg white Nasal discharge irritates nose Stopped nose Loss of smell and taste Cough with stitches in chest and bursting headache	Coldness Great weakness and weariness Depressed Weepy Wants sympathy, but annoyed by it Hoarseness Thirst for cold water Craves salt	About 10 A. M. Heat Consolation Noise Lying down Warm room	Lying on right side Open air Cold bath Going without regular meals
Nux vomica For Colds	Early stages Sneezing spells Runny nose during daytime, stopped up at night Sore throat	Irritable Chilly at slightest movement Feverish Extremely sensitive to noises and odors	Morning Cold air Open air	Evening Lying down Warmth Strong pressure on painful area Uninterrupted nap
For Coughs	Dry, teasing cough with sore throat and chest Cough with the sensation of something torn loose in chest Coughing spells ending in retching			
For Influenza	Cannot get warm Shivering, especially after drinking Cramping, griping pains causing urge to stool Nausea "Wants to and can't"; urge to stool, to vomit, but cannot			

COLDS, COUGHS, AND EARACHES

Remedy	Specific Indications	Guiding Symptoms	Worse From	Better From
Phosphorus For Coughs	Hard, dry, tickling cough "Clergyman's sore throat"; violent tickling in throat while speaking Racking cough with trembling Cough increases when talking or breathing cold air Pain in throat on coughing Heaviness as of a weight in chest Sweetish taste while coughing	Appears well despite high fever Colds go down into chest Chilly Thirsty for cold drinks, which are vomited as soon as warm in stomach Weak Anxious Hoarse Sweats at night	Evening Touch Warm food or drink Change of weather Getting wet in hot weather	Open air Sleep Cold food Cold
For Influenza	Nausea Burning pains in stomach, intestines			
Pulsatilla For Colds	"Ripe" cold Thick creamy yellow nasal discharge Eyelids stick together in morning Nose stuffed up at night and indoors Nose runs in open air Fever, but no thirst Lips chapped and peeling	Weepy Wants sympathy and attention Craves open air Dry mouth with lack of thirst	Toward evening Lying on left or on painless side Warmth Becoming overheated	Motion Open air Cold applications
For Cough	Paroxysms or coughing with gagging and choking Brings up thick yellow mucus Dry cough in evening; loose in morning Must sit up in bed to get relief Feeling of weight on chest			
For Earache	Red swollen external ear Thick yellow bland discharge Severe throbbing pain, worse at night Feels as if ears are stopped up			

COLDS, COUGHS, AND EARACHES

Remedy	Specific Indications	Guiding Symptoms	Worse From	Better From
Rumex For Coughs	Provoked by changing from warm to cold; breathing cold air Cough worse lying down, from pressing hand to throat Covers mouth to prevent inhaling cold air, which excites the cough Teasing cough, preventing sleep Violent, dry spasmodic cough Much tough, stringy mucus; urge to cough it up but cannot	Extremely sensitive to cold air Hoarse	Evening Inhaling cold air Uncovering Left side of chest	
Spongia For Coughs	Croupy cough; sounds like saw driven through a board Cough loud, dry, and barking Chest dry; no wheezing or rattling Throat sensitive to touch Difficult breathing, as if plug in throat Awakens with suffocative sensation, difficult breathing	Anxious Hoarse with soreness and burning Warm patient Exhaustion after slight exertion	Before midnight Talking Swallowing	Eating or drinking, especially warm drinks

7

Remedies for Stomach and Bowel Problems

JUDGING by television commercials, the Americans as a nation are obsessed with indigestion and "irregularity." Although millions of us spend hundreds of millions of dollars buying products to relieve these ailments ($223 million in one year for laxatives alone), people like yourself are seeking other ways. You are mistrustful of over-the-counter drugs that may worsen the situation, cause side effects, and quickly become habit forming You're learning about homeopathic remedies that support the body's natural self-regulatory functions and thus safely bring aid and comfort when minor problems occur, whether from stress, a restaurant meal, or a night on the town. If you're continually experiencing one upset after another, however, you would be wise to seek homeopathic care. The constitutional remedy, being suited to the individual's entire being, will not only put an end to recurring stomach and bowel complaints, but will give the person increased vitality and a sense of well-being.

INDIGESTION

"A meal a minute... fast take-out... the minute chef..." A stranger to American culture observing our commercial eating places might conclude that eating requires a stopwatch. Many of us follow the same pattern at home. The evening meal may be interrupted by phone calls, the pressure of parent-teacher association meetings. Singles frequently gulp a meal en route to an evening engagement.

If your frantic schedule is giving you indigestion, resolve to cut out the non-essentials. If you're still troubled by stomach distress, consider the following remedies, and choose one that fits you and your symptoms.

Bryonia. Your stomach feels heavy after eating and is sensitive to touch. You have bitter risings and may vomit bile and water. You are thirsty for long drinks of cold water, but may vomit from warm drinks. The least movement makes your stomach feel worse.

Carbo vegetabilis. The plainest food disagrees with you and causes gas and belching about one-half hour after eating. Any indulgence causes a headache. You have an aversion to meat, milk, and fatty foods, a craving for fresh air, and need to loosen your belt after eating.

Chamomilla. An attack of indigestion follows a fit of anger and irritability. Your stomach is distended with gas and cramping in the abdomen; your mouth has a bitter taste. You have flushed cheeks and an aversion to warm drinks.

Ignatia. You are tense, nervous, excitable, sensitive, and crave food that doesn't agree with you. Indigestion is caused by eating after receiving bad news or shock. Symptoms are rumbling in the bowels, sour belching. You have a tendency to take deep breaths or sigh frequently.

Nux vomica. You're the hard-driving type who overindulges in food, coffee, liquor, or tobacco. Symptoms are heartburn, belching, bloating of abdomen a few hours after eating. You may also be constipated.

Pulsatilla. You are peevish and wake up in the morning feeling as if you have a stone in your stomach; your mouth is dry with a bad taste but you're not thirsty. You have some of the same symptoms as *Carbo veg.*—pain in the stomach a half hour after eating, aversion to fatty foods and to snug clothing around the abdomen.

BEYOND FIRST AID: Abdominal pain may be a warning of appendicitis or other more serious problems. Therefore, when such pain persists and especially when accompanied by slight fever, nausea, vomiting, or even loss of appetite, seek professional help.

NAUSEA AND VOMITING

Eating and drinking too much or eating contaminated food are some common causes of vomiting. The following remedies will help relieve this condition.

Antimonium crudum (antimony). Vomiting caused by eating to excess or eating an indigestible substance. Patient vomits right after eating or drinking; has a white-coated tongue

Arsenicum. Nausea, vomiting, and diarrhea caused by spoiled food especially bad meat or watery fruit. Burning pains in the stomach after eating are relieved by warm drinks.

Colocynthis (bitter cucumber). Agonizing pain in the abdomen causes the patient to double up. Pressure and warmth applied to the stomach ameliorate the situation.

Ipecac. Nausea, griping pains in the intestines, with or without vomiting. Nausea from looking at moving objects, or reading in a moving vehicle. Tongue is clean, even though stomach is disordered.

Nux vomica. "Wants to and can't." This is a keynote of *Nux* whether the condition involves vomiting, moving bowels, or urinating. The patient is wakeful after 3 A.M., falls asleep toward morning, and awakens feeling wretched.

Phosphorus. Great thirst for cold water, which is vomited as soon as it becomes warm in the stomach. This remedy is also helpful in serious cases involving vomiting of blood.

Veratrum album. Patient alternates between vomiting and diarrhea. Cold sweat breaks out on the forehead, perhaps all over the body. Collapse is possible. Other symptoms are cramps in extremities and continued retching.

GAS

If you are not digesting your food properly, air or gas forms in the stomach and intestines. This can cause abdominal pain, bloating, rumbling, belching, and passing gas—and a good deal of embarrassment.

Like indigestion, gas is usually the result of eating too fast or eating while emotionally upset. Some people are also air swallowers; they "eat" air while talking or eating.

The digestive system is a marvelously synchronized effort, and each of its parts plays a distinct role in the process. If we don't chew our food thoroughly, the stomach, having no teeth, cannot break the food into small enough pieces to allow digestive juices to penetrate thoroughly, and thus the food passes into the intestines with its central portions undigested. Some of this undigested food will ferment, causing unpleasant-smelling intestinal gas and discomfort.

The following homeopathic remedies will help relieve this condition:

Carbo veg. The stomach fills up with gas no matter what you eat, resulting in repeated belching.

China. The stomach feels full of gas that won't come up or go down. The person's midsection feels distended.

Lycopodium. This is a feeling of fullness even before you finish eating or after a light meal. Belt feels too tight and there is rumbling gas and discharge.

COMMONSENSE MEASURES: Some of the foods that are commonly believed to cause gas are onions, cooked cabbage, raw apples, baked beans, and cucumbers. If any of these foods, or others, affect you this way, eliminate them from your diet.

No remedy, homeopathic or otherwise, should be taken regularly. If you are frequently troubled with stomach disorders, resolve to change your eating habits. Chew your food thoroughly; to be well absorbed, food must be broken into digestible particles in the mouth and mixed with the digestive enzymes that are in the saliva. If you must eat on the run, choose easily digested foods such as cottage cheese or curd.

Sip a cold drink—don't gulp. The lining of the stomach is well supplied with blood vessels; a large swallow of cold liquid can chill the stomach and cause it to go into spasm.

Another commonsense rule: Don't eat when you're not hungry, or when angry or overtired. You may have noticed that a dog will refuse food when frightened or exhausted from a chase. When you're tired, your stomach shares your fatigue; relax for at least a quarter hour before eating.

Antacids Are Antihealth

If, now and then, you get "off your feed," as one of my former patients expresses it, don't be brainwashed into taking one of the heavily advertised antacids. As promised, antacids "neutralize" stomach acid, but in moderate amounts stomach acid is not a villain; it is necessary for digestion. During digestion, the complex structure of our foods is broken down into simpler substances that can be absorbed and used by the body. Stomach acid kills or inactivates many germs which are in our food, so it is desirable to have *some* acid in the stomach.

Neutralizing acid also has an undesirable side effect: acid rebound, which means increased secretions of stomach acid that may persist long after the antacid action has ended. Consequently, the stomach's acid-producing cells must work harder to keep up the acid supply, and the result is excess acid in the stomach.

Use of antacids has been linked to brucellosis infection, also called undulant fever. The disease can be contracted from drinking unpasteurized infected milk. In a medical article, Dr. Robert Steffen of the University of California warns travelers who may be eating unpasteurized dairy products against heavy use of antacids. Brucellae are highly susceptible to gastric acid, this medical researcher notes, and gastric hypoacidity (insufficient acid) has been linked with travelers' diarrhea as well as more serious conditions.

Like many allopathic drugs, antacids can be harmful. These products taken over a prolonged period can cause either constipation or diarrhea, accompanied by nausea. Sodium bicarbonate (baking soda), a major ingredient in antacids, may lead to stone formation in the urinary tract and may also contribute to recurrent bladder infections. Magnesium-containing antacids can produce severe reactions, including lethargy, coma, circulatory collapse, and respiratory paralysis. All antacids are dangerous for persons with high blood pressure, kidney disease, a history of urinary stones or gastrointestinal bleeding.

CONSTIPATION

The body's way of disposing of waste material, like all its functions, is a marvel of design. After food has been digested, the colon muscles contract in a wave action called peristalsis, which carries its contents toward the rectum. On the way, the colon absorbs excess liquid from the mass of substance that comes from the small intestine. If you have not drunk enough fluids, the stool becomes dry and difficult to evacuate.

Constipation isn't a "modern" problem. The ancient Egyptians used the *Aloe vera* plant as a purgative. North American Indians, when in need of a cathartic, brewed the leaves of the senna plant. Judging by the U.S TV commercials ($ 16.8 million spent each year on advertising laxatives), we are still making a cripple of our poor colon by taking laxatives. As stated in a British medical journal: "The long-term use of laxatives ultimately leads to increasing constipation and the resort to even stronger purges." Severe chronic constipation can cause the colon to distend and lose more and more of its ability to contract.

Constipation can arise from organic causes, such as narrowing of the bowel and obstruction from growths, but the vast majority of cases of constipation stem from easily modified causes. These are: (1) A diet lacking in fiber or fluids. (2) Lack of exercise. (3) Negative emotional states, such as nervous tension, worry, and anxiety, that inhibit peristalsis and relaxation of anal sphincters. Many people who are "regular" at home become constipated on a trip. (4) Ignoring the signal to move the bowels. (Don't forget such tried-and-true aids as hot prune juice or lemon juice in hot water one-half hour before breakfast.)

You can prevent constipation by changing the above habits, but if you need immediate relief from constipation, choose a homeopathic remedy that stimulates a return to normalcy. If you're "hooked" on laxatives, *Nux vomica* will help break the habit. Take a dose upon retiring, or, better still, a few hours before bedtime; *Nux* acts best when mind and body are at rest. A daily dose may be needed for several days, but do not substitute a *Nux* habit for your former laxative habit. If you require repeated doses over a long period of time, you are not curing constipation, merely relieving it, and you need constitutional treatment.

If it's painful to pass stool owing to rectal fissure (a crack in the lining of the rectum), *Sulphur* will help restore the rectum to normal condition. You may have ineffective urging to stool, with burning at the anus, alternating with diarrhea. Faeces are hard, dark, and dry, and there is a tendency to hemorrhoids.

If you have difficulty passing stool, although your stool is so soft and sticky that a bowel movement requires quantities of toilet paper, consider *Alumina*. Homeopathic provings of *Alumina* were done many years ago, and provers reported difficult passage of soft, sticky stools. Repeated ingestion of small amounts of aluminium can cause this symptom, so if you're using aluminium cooking ware, this may be the cause of your bowel problem.

A large, hard, and dry stool, dark as if burnt, may indicate a need for *Bryonia*. Stools are passed with great difficulty owing to diminished intestinal secretions and poor muscle one. The person is irritable and ill tempered. Children who are constipated often need *Bryonia*.

A keynote of *Natrum mur* is a hard, crumbly stool that causes rectal bleeding, smarting, and soreness. There is contraction of the anus, bleeding, and pain.

When there is no urge to defecate, consider *Graphites* (from the mineral, graphite). You may go for days without a bowel movement, and when it finally comes, it takes the form of round balls stuck together with mucus and painful to pass. Other symptoms are fissures, or cracks, in the rectal mucosa, and hemorrhoids that burn and itch. The anus aches after passage of stool and becomes sore from wiping. The person who needs *Graphites* is often gloomy and obese.

An indication for *Silica* is a "bashful" stool that starts out and goes back. This difficulty is due to an insufficient expulsive power of the rectum and spasmodic condition of the sphincter muscle that surrounds and contracts the anus. There is soreness about the anus and often oozing of mucus.

Laxatives Make Your Body "Lax"

Above all, avoid chronic use of laxatives. The two main types produce an artificial action to stimulate peristalsis. One type, the irritant stimulant, does so by irritating nerve endings in the wall of the colon. The other, the saline cathartic, withdraws moisture from the intestinal lining, and the large volume of fluid then stimulates peristalsis. Mineral oil, which lubricates the stool, thus facilitating evacuation, has the disadvantage of causing embarrassing leakage; continued use also cuts down on absorption of vitamins.

All laxatives, no matter how they work, are taking over a job that the body should be doing. Don't delude yourself that you're doing something "natural" by taking an herbal laxative. All laxatives, whether herbal or synthetic, cause a "lazy" bowel and are habit forming. In my experience, the person troubled with constipation must discontinue all laxatives and rely on commonsense measures aided by a homeopathic remedy, if needed, to restore normal bowel function. The bowel that has been whipped and tortured by harsh purgatives will naturally take a longer time to recover.

DIARRHEA

Diarrhea—frequent and excessive discharge of watery stools—is most often an acute condition caused by eating something unfamiliar to the body, perhaps food that is highly seasoned

STOMACH AND BOWEL PROBLEMS

or spoiled. The experience is unpleasant but next time it occurs, consider what an efficient way this is for your body to get rid of an undesirable substance.

The following homeopathic remedies will help relieve the miseries of diarrhea without interfering with its cleansing action.

Arsenicum. The stomach feels heavy; patient experiences nausea and vomiting; there is a feeling of weakness. This comes from eating spoiled food or excessive amounts of any fruit, particularly melons. *Arsenicum* will not interfere with the discharge of toxic substances but will bring about order in the irritated intestinal tract so that diarrhea is no longer needed.

Cuprum arsenicosum (arsenate of copper). Symptoms are burning, cramping, colicky pains in the lower bowels, accompanied by vomiting and diarrhea, with cramps and sensation of collapse.

This remedy proved helpful recently for a young man who rushed into the office without an appointment and begged to see me. "I'm running late," I explained, but after hearing his plight, I relented. He had eaten a Mexican dinner the night before and, since early morning, had suffered diarrhea and weakness. He had taken *Arsenicum*, which had not helped. In the last hour, he had developed severe cramping, which indicated *Cuprum ars*. After taking the remedy, he lay down on the examining table, and within fifteen minutes, the cramping had subsided. At my suggestion, he rested another half hour and then left, feeling recovered.

Gelsemium. Diarrhea from anticipation of even an enjoyable social engagement, or from fear of an ordeal. Loose movements may also follow a fright.

Podophyllum (May apple). Diarrhea—yellow watery stools that are squirted out—occurs in the early morning or after eating. Patient may have cramps that are relieved by warmth and bending double. After having a bowel movement, patient experiences a weak feeling in the abdomen and feels "all in."

Sulphur. Stools are changeable; sometimes they are yellow and watery, other times slimy, with undigested food. Urgent need to defecate drives the patient out of bed first thing in the morning.

Veratrum album. Symptoms are similar to *Arsenicum* but, in addition, patient experiences a cold sweat and feels on the verge of collapse.

I have seen *Veratrum alb.* work dramatically in the case of a young woman named Ellen going through the trauma of divorce. Ellen called me one day. "I have to appear in court this morning," she said weakly, "and I'm having diarrhea and throwing up at the same time." She was also in a cold sweat, she said, and felt as if she were going to collapse any minute. I told her to take *Veratrum alb.* and call me in a half hour. At that time, she reported that the vomiting and diarrhea had stopped, and she felt strong enough to face the ordeal ahead.

COMMONSENSE MEASURES: Restore fluid balance in the body by taking plenty of liquids such as water, tea, and clear soups. Avoid milk. When diarrhea eases off, add tea and toast, and follow with a bland diet.

BEYOND FIRST AID: The chief danger in diarrhea is that the person may become dehydrated, or if the condition becomes chronic, that it can lead to anemia and malnutrition. Should diarrhea persist more than a few days, consult your doctor.

If your diarrhea is severe and you do not have the necessary homeopathic remedy, a kaolin-pectin mixture is a helpful temporary measure. This combination prevents absorption of bacterial toxins by forming a film on the intestinal wall and itself absorbing some of these toxins.

Paregoric, a form of opium, paralyzes the action of the intestinal waves (peristalsis), and thus opposes the body's efforts to expel toxic matter. *Do not use.*

HEMORRHOIDS (Piles)

A hemorrhoid is an enlarged or varicose vein in the region of the rectum, an extremely sensitive area. These veins can become so distended that they protrude, rupture, and bleed. According to some estimates, one-half of all adult Americans suffer from hemorrhoids.

Fortunately, homeopathy can help this common affliction and has been doing so for over 150 years. To relieve painful hemorrhoids, take a sitz bath—a warm tub bath—for ten to fifteen minutes, at least twice a day. Then apply *Aesculus* and *Hamamelis* ointment. *Aesculus* is homeopathically prepared from the horse chestnut (*Aesculus hippocastanum*), and *Hamamelis virginica* is made from the witch hazel shrub. This preparation relieves itching, pain, and inflammation, and aids healing.

Internal homeopathic remedies (tablets or powders), when indicated, will also relieve discomfort and promote healing. The person needing *Aesculus* experiences a burning sensation in the rectum, a dull ache in the lower back, and shooting pains upward. The lining of the rectum seems swollen and obstructs the passageway. The hemorrhoids look like a bunch of purple grapes.

British homeopath, Dr. A. C. Gordon Ross, in his book, *Homeopathic Green Medicine*, writes: "This is one of the best homeopathic remedies for piles, and I have gained whole families as lifelong patients just because a few powders of *Aesculus hippocastanum* cured grandfather's piles in a week."

Arnica, which heals damaged tissue, is useful for hemorrhoids that develop after childbirth. During childbirth, the pressure of the baby's head may cause trauma to tissues. I've seen tremendously swollen, angry-looking hemorrhoids in a new mother respond to *Arnica*.

Collinsonia (a stone root) has the sensation of sticks in the rectum; the patient is usually constipated. When *Nitric acid* is indicated, hemorrhoids feel like needles or splinters in the rectum. *Nux vomica* is characterized by itching; the hemorrhoids are better from cool bathing. *Sulphur* is the remedy for itching and burning around the anus made worse by bathing, an unusual symptom for hemorrhoids. The condition is also worse from rubbing and standing, and worse at night.

On occasion, a remedy not indicated for hemorrhoids may prove helpful for that condition. One of my patients, a farmer, strained his back and I gave him *Arnica*. A few days later, his wife telephoned: "Was there anything in those pills for piles? My husband has had that trouble for years, and he's so much better since you treated his back."

COMMONSENSE MEASURES: Hemorrhoids are generally caused by straining during bowel movements, which pushes out the veins. If your hemorrhoids are due to constipation, see the list of causes mentioned in the section on "Constipation" and try to correct those habits. In addition, a warm bath several times a day will help to relax the muscles that encircle the anus.

BEYOND FIRST AID: Severe pain may mean that you have a thrombosed hemorrhoid (blood clot). You will obtain instant relief from a minor surgical procedure in which the surgeon nicks the skin of the vein causing the clot to "pop out." If there is rectal bleeding, check with your physician to make sure there is nothing more serious than hemorrhoids.

QUICK REFERENCE CHART

STOMACH AND BOWEL PROBLEMS

Dosage: Two tablets taken 3 or 4 times a day—or, when pain is severe, every 30 minutes to 1 hour Decrease frequency of dosage as patient improves; discontinue when improvement is well established.

If you are under the care of a homeopathic physician, *do not take any remedies for acute illnesses without checking with your doctor.*

Remedy	Indications	Worse From	Better From
Aesculus For Hemorrhoids	Burning sensation Dull ache in lower back Lining of rectum seems swollen and obstructs passageway Look like a bunch of purple grapes Sharp shooting pains upward	Any motion Awakening Moving bowels Standing Walking	Cool, open air

Aesculus and Hamamelis Ointment For Hemorrhoids	Relieves:
	  Itching
	  Pain
	  Inflammation		

Alumina For Constipation	Itching and burning at anus Stool hard, dry, knotty, covered with mucus Stool clayey, clings to anus Much straining to pass even a soft stool	Afternoon Time to time Eating potatoes	Damp weather
Antimonium crudum For Vomiting	Occurs on eating or drinking From indigestible substance From overeating Constant belching White-coated tongue	Evening Acids Washing Water Wine	During rest Open air
Arnica For Hemorrhoids	Following childbirth	Least touch Motion Rest	Lying down with head low
Arsenicum General	Cannot bear sight or smell of food Thirsty for small, frequent sips Burning pains Restless	Right side Cold drinks Food Cold	Head elevated Heat warm drinks

STOMACH AND BOWEL PROBLEMS

Remedy	Indication	Worse From	Better From
Arsenicum For Diarrhea	After eating or drinking Followed by great weakness Offensive odor Painful cramping Stools, bloody, watery, or dark-colored Heaviness in stomach	Highly seasoned food Spoiled foods Too much watery fruit	
For Vomiting	After eating or drinking With nausea and retching Vomiting of blood, bile, brown-black mucus mixed with blood, or green mucus Stomach seems raw Followed by extreme exhaustion		
Bryonia General	Ill-tempered Irritable Thirsty for long drinks of cold water Stitching, tearing pains	Morning Eating Motion Touch Warm drinks	Lying on painful side Eating Firm pressure Rest
For Constipation	In children Difficult passing from poor muscle tone Diminished intestinal secretions Large, hard dry stool, as if burnt		
For Indigestion	Bitter risings Stomach feels heavy after eating Stomach sensitive to touch Vomiting of bile or water Vomiting of warm drinks		
Carbo vegetabilis General	Coldness A chilly patient with air hunger	Evening Lying down Wine	Belching Fanning Cold
For Indigestion	Aversion to meat, milk, and fatty foods Cramping pain causing person to bend double Gas and belching $\frac{1}{2}$ hour after eating Simplest food disagrees, causes gas Wants clothing loose around abdomen Abdomen bloated with gas		

STOMACH AND BOWEL PROBLEMS

Remedy	Indications	Worse From	Better From
Chamomilla General	Anxious tossing Extreme restlessness One cheek hot, the other pale and cold Snappish; asks for something then flings it away Oversensitive to pain	Heat Anger Open air Night	Warm wet weather
For Indigestion	Abdomen distended with gas Bitter taste Cramping in abdomen Following fit of anger or irritability Sweats after eating or drinking		
China For Indigestion	Gas won't come up or down Belching gives no relief Stomach feels full, heavy	Night Slightest touch Every other day Eating Drafts	Bending double Hard pressure Open air Warmth
Collinsonia For Hemorrhoids	Sensation of sharp sticks in rectum Chronic, painful bleeding Constipation	Slightest excitement Cold	Heat
Colocynthis For Vomiting	Severe, cutting abdominal pain Patient doubles up from pain	Anger Indignation	Pressure Warmth
Cuprum arsenicosum For Diarrhea	Sense of collapse Abdomen tense, hot, tender Intense burning cramping pain in lower bowels, abdomen, fingers, calves, feet Stools slimy and brown Vomiting	Touch	Night Lying on affected side Pressure Warmth
Gelsemium General	Chills up and down back Heaviness of limbs and eyelids Trembling	10 A.M. Thinking of ailment Anticipation	Bending forward Profuse urination Continued motion
For Diarrhea	Cream-colored or tea-green From emotional excitement, fright, bad news Involuntary Painless		

STOMACH AND BOWEL PROBLEMS

Remedy	Indications	Worse From	Better From
Graphites General	Chilly Gloomy Obese	Night During and after menses Warmth	Eating Hot foods and drink
For Constipation	Anus aches after stool Anus sore from wiping Itching of anus No urge to defecate Stool: large round balls stuck together with tough slimy mucus		
For Hemorrhoids	Burn Itch		
Ignatia General	Excitable Nervous Sensitive Frequent sighing Takes deep breaths Tense	Morning Motion Brandy Coffee Strong odors Tobacco smoke	Lying on painful side Warmth Walking
For Indigestion	After receiving bad news or shock Craves food that doesn't agree Rumbling in bowels Sour belching		
Ipecac For Vomiting	Constant and continual nausea Clean tongue Great flow of saliva Griping pains in intestines Preceded by nausea	Lying down Veal	Slightest motion
Lycopodium For Indigestion	Feeling of fullness even before finishing eating or after light meal Bloating, distension of stomach and abdomen; must loosen clothing Rumbling of gas Discharge of flatus Incomplete, burning belchings rise only partially to throat, burn there for hours Heartburn Craving for sweets	Right side 4 to 8 P.M. Cold drinks Heat or warm room	After midnight Warm food or drink Motion Getting cold Uncovering

STOMACH AND BOWEL PROBLEMS

Remedy	Indications	Worse From	Better From
Natrum muriaticum General	Hates fuss Irritable Weepy	Noise Warm room Lying down At seashore Mental exertion Heat	Open air Cold bathing Going without regular meals Tight clothing
For Constipation	Anus bleeding, contracted, torn Burning pains after stool Irregular, dry, crumbly stool		
Nitric acid For Hemorrhoids	Bleed easily Feel as if needles in rectum Great pain after stool; lasts for hours	Evening and night During sweat On waking Walking	Riding in a car

Nux Vomica
General
	Hard-driving personality
	Irritable
	Oversensitive to outside stimuli:
	  noise, odors, light, etc.
	"Wants to and can't"
		Morning
		After eating
		Cold
		Narcotics
		Spices
		Stimulants
		Open air
			Evening
			Strong pressure
			Uninterrupted
			  nap
			Warmth

For Constipation	To help relieve the laxative habit Frequent and ineffectual desire for stool "Something left behind"		
For Hemorrhoids	Itching Relieved by cool bathing		
For Indigestion	Belching: sour, bitter Bloating of abdomen few hours after eating Heartburn Overindulgence in food, coffee, liquor, tobacco		
For Vomiting	With nausea Much retching		
Phosphorus For Vomiting	Of blood Of food scarcely swallowed Great thirst for cold water, vomited as soon as warm Sour taste and belching	Evening Touch Warm food or drink	Lying on right side Cold Cold food Open air Sleep
Podophyllum For Diarrhea	Followed by weakness in abdomen Much colic Stool yellow, watery, with jelly-like mucus Flatulence Gushing, profuse Painless Offensive odor Gurgling in abdomen, then sudden, profuse diarrhea While bathing or being washed	Early morning Teething Hot weather	

STOMACH AND BOWEL PROBLEMS

Remedy	Indications	Worse From	Better From
Pulsatilla General	Dry mouth Thirstless Peevish Weeps easily	Twilight Lying on left or painless side Rich, fatty food	Motion Open air Cold food and drinks, though not thirsty
For Indigestion	Averse to fat food, warm food and drink Belching Dry mouth with bitter taste Flatulence Heartburn Stomach pain about an hour after eating Wants clothing loose around abdomen Weight as if stone in stomach, especially on awakening	After eating Warm room	Cold applications
Silica General	Chilly Anxious Yielding	Morning During menses Cold	Warmth
For Constipation	"Bashful" stool; starts out and goes back Much straining, but cannot expel		
Sulphur For Constipation	Burning anus with itching Pain at stool from rectal fissure Ineffective urging alternating with diarrhea "Something left behind" Stool hard, dry, dark Stool large and painful, held back from pain	Bathing Standing Warmth of bed	Lying on right side
For Hemorrhoids	Burning Itching		
For Diarrhea	Changeable stools; one yellow and watery, another slimy, undigested food Morning diarrhea, drives patient out of bed		
Veratrum album General	Coldness Cold sweat Cold sweat on forehead Collapse	Drinking Least motion	Warmth
For Diarrhea	Copious Exhaustion Painful Followed by great weakness Forcibly evacuated Watery		
For Vomiting	Alternating with diarrhea Cramps in extremities Profuse vomiting and nausea Thirst for cold water, vomited as soon as swallowed		

8

A Happier Baby with Homeopathic Care

"My baby was screaming with colicky pains. Living in the wilds of South Dakota, I had no one to turn to. We had no phone, my husband had the car. Our nearest neighbor was five miles away."

Jane had many such incidents to relate about their first baby. Fortunately, Jane knew what to do for colic and other acute infant ailments. She and her husband Tom had studied homeopathy before moving to South Dakota. They had consulted a colleague of mine in Indianapolis and equipped themselves with a home remedy kit. Today the couple have three children (ages four, five, and nine), and live in an equally remote area in Minnesota. In winter, they're snowbound for days at a time. The other day, contemplating this chapter, I called Jane and asked her which remedies had been most helpful to her when her trio were babies.

"*Aconite, Belladonna, Chamomilla,*" she said, referring to what Dr. John H. Clarke, an English homeopath, called the ABCs of childhood. They have brought peace and comfort to countless babies without exposing them to the risk of allergic sensitivity or drug side effects. "When Jane, our oldest, had colic, she was so cranky I didn't know what to do with her. I gave her a dose of *Chamomilla*, and the cramps went away.

"When my kids were teething, they often ran a fever," Jane continued. "Tommy's face would be so red and hot it felt like fire. *Belladonna* worked like a charm. But when Jennifer, our youngest, was teething, only one cheek was red and warm, and the other was cool. And she was so cranky I knew she must need *Chamomilla*. I gave her a dose, and she was fine."

As for *Aconite*, whose mental symptoms include fear of death, Jane described an incident in which the entire family benefited from this remedy.

"We had just moved to South Dakota when a tornado whipped by. We ran out and hid in a ditch knee-deep in mud. We were scared to death—we couldn't talk—nothing would come out. My oldest daughter was particularly upset; she was stuttering, her eyes wide with fear. As soon as we got back to the house, I gave everybody a dose of *Aconite*, which calmed us all down."

Now you may not be as geographically isolated as Jane and her husband, but in our impersonal urban society, a new parent can suffer from a terrible sense of isolation. Often, there is no aunt or grandmother nearby to offer advice or take over the baby when you feel

A HAPPIER BABY

as if you're on your last legs. Even though you may have your own physician, babies have a way of getting sick in the middle of the night, and you may not want to bother your doctor unless you believe it's a real emergency.

In this chapter you will learn about a host of remedies to enable you to cope with your baby's acute ailments. But don't interpret this as a go-ahead to give your baby a remedy for each slight discomfort. Although a homeopathic remedy has no side effects, each dose is a signal to the defense mechanism. Bombarding the system with one signal after another is bound to result in confusion. Reserve your homeopathic remedy for those times when it is really needed.

Don't expect to be an instant prescriber. As Jane expressed it, "If you're going to use homeopathy, you must educate yourself, be willing to read, learn the proper uses of a remedy. And the rewards are worth it. With my knowledge of homeopathy, I never feel helpless when the children get sick."

Babies are generally healthy and seldom need medicine of any kind. There are times, however, when a baby is cross and miserable and this upsets the entire household. Exhausted, red-eyed parents wonder if they can face the next day. It is immensely comforting to know that you can select a safe and effective remedy that will not only relieve your baby, but deal with the problem that is making the child so unhappy.

POOR SLEEPING HABITS

If your baby isn't sleeping well, then usually nothing goes right. You're exhausted and short-tempered. So the sooner you can determine the cause of sleeplessness, the better. If your baby is sleepless from colic, see the section on colic in this chapter. If the problem is teething, the section on teething should be helpful.

Sometimes a baby's poor sleeping habits are caused by overeating, indigestion, too many bedcoverings, or too warm a room. Investigate these causes, all of which are easy to remedy. Another factor is the well-known separation anxiety that most babies display at some time. When you disappear, your baby doesn't know whether you are coming back, or, for that matter, if you still exist and may howl just to make sure that you're still around.

For many years, parents have given infants phenobarbital or other sedatives. These drugs will put a baby to sleep, but have no effect on the underlying problem. And they carry a high risk. An overdose of a sedative can be fatal.

BEYOND FIRST AID: If instead of sleeping, your baby rocks the crib across the floor or rhythmically bangs his or her head against the crib side or mattress, the child may be displaying signs of intracranial tension. This condition is usually an after effect of the birth trauma. During the birth process, the skull bones overlap a little, thus reducing the size of the head to ease the passage down the birth canal. As the baby's head emerges and the pressure is released, the bones usually settle into their proper position. Sometimes, however, they do not align perfectly.

Robert C. Fulford, D.O., now retired, has been a pioneer in the techniques of cranial osteopathy. Dr. Fulford explains that the circulation of the vital cerebrospinal fluid, which bathes the brain and nerve centers, can be impeded by faulty relationships in the position of the cranial bones. Gentle manipulation of the skull bones can release the tension and greatly improve functioning of the baby's whole body.

ALLERGIES

Allergy problems often crop up during the baby's first or second year. Babies are often allergic to cow's milk, house dust, or dog hair. An allergy may be signaled by dark rings under the eyes, sometimes called the "allergic shiner"; by a perpetual cold; or by such diverse symptoms as colic, diarrhea, or a skin rash.

The standard medical treatment for an allergy is to discover and remove the offending substance. For example, if the culprit is house dust, exposure to dust is reduced and repeated injections of a series of varying dilutions of house dust are given. This treatment is called desensitization. Sometimes it relieves symptoms, sometimes not. If the symptoms persist, the treatment must be continued indefinitely.

On the other hand, a homeopathic remedy will not only relieve the symptoms but also put the system back in balance—thereby removing the allergy. For this, constitutional prescribing is necessary.

BEYOND FIRST AID: If you suspect that your baby has an allergy, seek professional homeopathic help. Using a home remedy you might remove a symptom, but in doing so, obscure the indications on which a homeopathic physician prescribes. You can, of course, try to figure out the cause of the allergy and remove it, but this is a temporary measure.

COLDS

A baby with a cold is so defenseless. The child is uncomfortable, can't eat and breathe at the same time, and hasn't learned how to breathe through the mouth. Homeopathic remedies can relieve this discomfort and frustration.

In general, dosage is two tablets three times a day. Some conditions call for more frequent repetition, others less. The more severe the illness, the more frequently a dose is needed. As a careful observer and prescriber, you will learn to suit the dosage to the needs of the baby. Remember, a homeopathic remedy is not like penicillin that you take four times a day for ten days. You are not trying to maintain a certain concentration of a drug in the blood stream, or to kill germs. You are trying to stimulate the defense mechanism so that your baby's body can heal itself without the use of a powerful drug.

We've already discussed *Aconite* as a remedy for sudden intense fear. But *Aconite*, like so many homeopathic remedies, has many uses. It's a good remedy for a cold that comes on suddenly, particularly after exposure to a cold wind or draft. Perhaps you've put the baby out in her carriage on a cold day, bundled up with plenty of covers so you know she's warm enough, but you don't realize how windy it is. Soon after, she comes down with a cold that quickly settles in her chest; there's a harsh sound to her breathing. Give her *Aconite*. She may need frequent repetition at first, sometimes hourly, if symptoms are severe, but not more often than needed to keep her improving.

A *Belladonna* cold comes on suddenly, too, often after exposing the head to cold or washing the hair. You put your baby to bed one evening and he's perfectly well; that night he wakens flushed, restless, his skin hot to the touch. He blinks and whimpers when you turn on the light; if you look closely, you'll see that his pupils are dilated, and, therefore, he's more sensitive to light. This could be a sore throat or the beginning of a head cold. If your baby shows these key symptoms—red face, hot skin, with cold extremities and restlessness—then *Belladonna* is the remedy.

Thus far, we've talked about two remedies, *Aconite* and *Belladonna*, for colds that come on suddenly. The *Gelsemium* cold sneaks up on its victim. When you put your baby to bed, he's quieter than usual and seems lethargic; he has no fever so you decide he's just tired. In the morning he looks droopy, including his eyes, which are heavylidded. He has a low-grade fever but doesn't want anything to drink. During the day he may run a higher temperature and seem generally uncomfortable. Feel his pulse—you'll find it soft and flowing in contrast to that of the child who needs *Belladonna*, whose pulse is hard and bounding. (It's a good idea to feel the pulse when your baby's well, so that you'll become familiar with the variations caused by illness.)

Pulsatilla is for the "ripe" cold, with thick, creamy, bland mucus. The other day I had a call from a patient whose baby had this type of cold. "He's weepy, he wants to be petted, and he's so changeable; one minute he seems well, the next, he's miserable." I asked her, "Is he better inside or when you take him out?" "Oh, he's much better outside; he gets stuffy as soon as I bring him in." One of the symptoms of *Pulsatilla* is a craving for open air. This in itself is not enough to prescribe on, but, in this case, all the symptoms pointed to *Pulsatilla*.

Sometimes a cold sounds worse than it is. I recently saw a six-month-old girl who had a rattling sound when she breathed or coughed; her mother was afraid that she had a chest infection. I examined her and found that her lungs were clear. The rattling sound was caused by mucus rolling back and forth in the larger air passages. The baby was sweaty, extremely irritable, with a constant discharge of yellow mucus from one nostril that ran down her lip. All these symptoms indicated *Hepar sulph.*, which cleared up the condition in two days.

Hepar sulphuris is an excellent medicine for babies with a cold, and belongs in every household remedy kit. The baby who needs *Hepar sulph.* is apt to be sweaty, cough readily, and have rattling breathing. *Hepar* has an unusual weather indication: The patient is better in damp weather and worse from dry, cold weather.

If your baby has a sore throat and swollen neck glands, think of *Mercurius vivus*. Your child can't tell you about a sore throat, but you can probably detect the swollen glands. Lightly touch each side of the neck; you may feel an enlargement of the lymph nodes, which are little filters that strain out the impurities of the blood from the affected areas. The baby who needs *Mercurius* is sweaty, smells sick, and may have diarrhea along with the cold. The child is worse at night, apt to be trembly, and may drool more than usual.

Mercurius is made from potentized pure mercury, or quick silver; it is used to treat both minor and serious diseases. Mercury in the thermometer is insoluble in water. Hahnemann, the founder of homeopathy, transformed the metal into an active medicinal agent by grinding it for hours in a mortar (trituration), with lactose, which is milk sugar.

The *Bryonia* baby, that is, the baby who needs *Bryonia* due to a cold, has a dry stuffy nose and dry lips. She's irritable, cries for something and then refuses it, and hates to be moved. She's extremely thirsty; you offer her water and she slurps it up. She's apt to be constipated with hard, dry stools. The *Bryonia* cough is distinctive; unlike the loose rattling-mucus cough of *Hepar*, it's a dry, harsh sound. Keep this cough in mind when you consider *Bryonia*, but try not to prescribe on just one symptom. A homeopathic prescription is like a three-legged stool; it can't rest on one leg, or symptom, alone.

Dulcamara has the keynote symptom—hypersensitivity to cold and especially wet, cold weather. So, if the day the two of you were caught in the rain your baby got chilled and developed a cold, consider this remedy. *Solanum dulcamara* is bittersweet or woody nightshade, a climbing shrub. It has been used as a medicine since the thirteenth century. Hahnemann, in 1811, proved it on himself and others and found that he and his colleagues suffered especially in cold, wet weather.

Last, we have *Nux vomica*, a polychrest for many common ailments. The *Nux* baby has sniffles; his nose drips in the daytime, is stuffy at night and out-of-doors. He may do a lot of burping, and is constipated; he'll strain to pass a stool but with little result. He is often worse at four in the morning.

As you can see, prescribing for a cold is not an instant procedure; it takes time and thought, and, even then, you can make mistakes. My biggest "goof," in respect to colds, was the occasion of my visit to the Himalayan Institute in Chicago. Making rounds with its medical director, Dr. Rudolph Ballentine, and his associate, Dr. Dennis K. Chernin, we examined a child with a chronic cold. The two doctors then asked me what remedy I would suggest, and I said "*Gelsemium*." The child seems so lethargic, I explained. He's heavy-lidded, has a slight watery nasal discharge, and is'nt thirsty. I could tell that Rudy didn't agree with me, but he was very polite about it. "Let's give him a dose of *Gelsemium*," he said, "and we'll see how he is tomorrow." The next day, to my chagrin, the child was no better. The two doctors then recommended *Mercurius*, which I hadn't considered at all. It was obviously the right remedy; the child improved dramatically the following day. (For further discussion of colds, see chapter 7.)

BEYOND FIRST AID: What appears to be a cold may sometimes be an allergy. In this case, seek professional homeopathic help.

EARACHES

The baby that develops an ear infection is apt to have a shrill, piercing cry. You can usually tell where it hurts; the infant tosses its head about and beats or pulls at an ear. Its face is probably flushed and its ears are red. If the onset is sudden, if the child is restless, and, particularly, if the ear in question is the right one, then *Belladonna* is your remedy. *Belladonna*, inexplicably, is a right-sided remedy. We know this from the experience of provers testing *Belladonna*; nearly all their symptoms were on the right sides.

Other remedies that are useful for babies with earaches:

Aconite. Sudden onset after exposure to cold wind or draft.

Chamomilla. Wild with pain, extremely irritable; wants to be carried about and is worse from warmth. Sometimes one cheek is red, the other pale.

Dulcamara. Onset after change to cold, damp weather; worse at night.

Ferrum phos. Like *Belladonna*, baby has a flushed face, is sensitive to touch and noise and hates being jarred. But symptoms come on gradually instead of suddenly. This remedy is useful at the beginning of an earache, when *Belladonna* doesn't fit.

Hepar sulph. Sticking pain going from throat into ears; sensitive to draft, worse from the least draft or cold.

Magnesia phos. Earache is worse on the right side, worse from cold and at night. Earache feels better from warmth and pressure.

Pulsatilla. Earache is worse from heat. Baby feels better in the open air; is thirstless, weepy, and wants lots of attention.

Verbascum thapsus is a little-known remedy that has left-sided symptoms. It is made from the mullein plant, which is still used by herbalists for its soothing properties. Think of *Verbascum* for an earache in the left ear. Baby is hoarse, and may have a deep-toned cough.

COLIC

Colic is a general term meaning spasmodic pain in the abdomen. In the infant, it usually means a digestive upset as evidenced by the baby's crying, doubling up as if in pain, and passing intestinal gas with temporary relief. This is not a serious problem—most infants outgrow it by three to four months—but while baby is suffering, it's distressing to all. Fortunately, homeopathy can help.

Debbie, at seven months, was brought to me by her grandmother, who cared for her while Debbie's mother worked. Debbie had been given a series of formulas since birth, none of which had agreed with her, then put on solid food. As her grandmother related, she was very cranky and would constantly double up and scream with gas pains. "The only thing that relieved her was my putting my hand on her little stomach."

The keynote for *Colocynthis* is that the child's abdomen feels better from firm pressure. One of the great prescribers, Dr. F.B. Nash, said, "No remedy produces more severe colic than this one, and no remedy cures more promptly." I gave Debbie *Colocynthis*, and, after a few days, she began to digest her food better; the colicky pains disappeared. Within two weeks, she could tolerate any foods offered.

There's another fine remedy for colic that was a big help to me as a mother. Our daughter Anne, at two months, was miserable and cranky. Almost every evening she would draw up her knees and cry. It soothed her if I held her on my shoulder or laid her over my lap on a hot-water bottle. We gave her *Magnesia phosphorica*, which quickly relieved her discomfort.

Why this particular remedy for colic? One of the strong indications for *Magnesia phos.* is relief from warmth and from gentle pressure on the abdomen. The keynote for *Colocynthis* is relief from firm pressure and doubling up.

The colicky baby who needs *Bryonia* presents a different picture. I recently received a phone call from one of my young mothers. Her baby was screaming with a bellyache, but she couldn't do anything to soothe her. "She doesn't want to be carried," she said. "She asks for a drink, then doesn't want it. When I put a hot-water bottle on her stomach, she screamed and pushed it away." Those symptoms fit *Bryonia*—irritable and worse from the least movement or jarring; can't stand to be moved.

The colicky baby who needs *Chamomilla* is also a trial to a parent. As one mother described it: "He wants to be carried constantly but that doesn't help. He cries for water, then doesn't want it. He whines for a toy, then throws it away. He's impossible!" Besides being extremely cranky and "impossible," the *Chamomilla* baby often has one red cheek, the other pale.

As an experienced homeopath said: "You cannot please the child who needs *Chamomilla* —you cannot soothe him. Just give him his remedy, and his disposition will improve."

DIARRHEA

Diarrhea can be a serious condition in an infant. A greater proportion of an infant's body weight is water as compared with an adult's. If diarrhea is copious and continues for any length of time, the baby loses proportionately too much body fluid and becomes dehydrated. Dehydration, which is loss of fluid from tissues and blood, can damage circulation. If your baby has several watery stools in one day, this doesn't mean she is dehydrating, but be alert to this possibility.

Here is a list of remedies that will help different types of diarrhea:

Aconite. After exposure to cold wind.

Arsenicum album. Diarrhea resulting from spoiled food or too much fruit. Frequent dark, offensive stools; restlessness, thirst for small sips of water, weakness.

Chamomilla. Greenish slimy stools during teething.

Colocynthis. Severe cramping; when every bite of food is followed by rush of diarrhea.

Nux vomica. Diarrhea resulting from overfeeding, especially if the baby strains without result, or passes only a small quantity with each attempt.

Podophyllin. Watery, undigested stools, forcibly expelled; immediately upon eating or drinking or being bathed; occurs most often in early morning.

VOMITING

If your baby spits up after every feeding, this is usually nothing to worry about. During meal time, he may fill his stomach but continue drinking to satisfy his sucking needs. If he drinks too much, he will spit up the excess.

Spitting up works like an overflow mechanism in a sink. This is different from vomiting, in which the contents of the stomach are heaved up with some degree of force. If this occurs, first seek the cause. Perhaps he has eaten some food, or nonfood, that disagrees with him. (Almost every family has a story about a baby ingesting some inedible; in ours, it was the cover of his father's law journal.) If the vomiting, however, signifies the beginning of an acute illness, then the right remedy will relieve the baby's discomfort and speed recovery.

Ipecac, best known of the vomiting remedies, is used as syrup of ipecac in first-aid treatment to induce vomiting when a child has swallowed poison. A homeopath, knowing that what a drug causes it can cure, uses potentized *Ipecac* to check uncontrollable vomiting or persistent nausea.

Here is a list of the remedies to consider for vomiting:

Aconite From nervous upset or fright.

Arsenicum. From spoiled food or eating too much fruit.

Bryonia. From rich or fatty food; baby is irritable, wants to be left alone.

Ipecac. Especially after eating; persistent nausea with a clean tongue.

Phosphorus. Great thirst for cold water, which is vomited as soon as warm in the stomach.

DIAPER RASH

Why does your baby develop diaper rash while your neighbor, who launders diapers just as you do, has no such problem with her baby? This may be just another demonstration that no two babies are alike. Does your baby wear paper diapers? You might try another brand to see if it makes any difference. Or, plastic pants might cause, or aggravate, the condition. Waterproof pants prevent evaporation of body fluids, thus keeping the diaper area constantly moist, which encourages growth of germs. A better solution is the specially treated all-cotton diaper cover, available at better stores.

Let your baby crawl about with a bare bottom several times a day, confined to a safe area, of course. A quick tub soak between changes will also help. For a soothing and healing ointment, apply *Calendula* ointment, which has a lanolin base. In her book, *Homeopathy for the First Aider*, the late Dorothy Shepherd extols the virtues of *Calendula* ointment as a soothing and healing preparation. "It is of much greater value than the ubiquitous boracic, zinc, or calamine ointments," she writes. I agree with Dr. Shepherd. So often one of my mothers will bring in a baby with a sore bottom. "I've tried all the ointments but the rash doesn't clear up." She tries *Calendula* ointment and soon reports that the rash is gone.

TEETHING

"The little patient is cross, peevish, and whining, or obstinate and ugly. It is satisfied with nothing. It howls when denied something that it thinks it wants and strikes it angrily to the floor if it is proffered. When touched, or even when looked at, the child manifests its resentment by shrieks, whining, or angry cries. It is quiet only when carried about."

This is a description of a baby who needs *Chamomilla* during difficult teething. It jibes with my experience. A mother called me the other day. "I don't know what's the matter with Billy. He's so cranky—nothing pleases him. He wants to be carried, then cries to be put down. He wants a drink, then pushes it away." It sounded as if Billy were teething, since he chewed on his fist, drooled a lot, and had a slight fever.

I prescribed *Chamomilla*, two tablets every two hours, until he showed improvement. The next day, Billy's mother called me again. He had gone to sleep after the second dose and was his own cheerful self when he woke up.

The baby who needs *Belladonna* will be irritable but not as cross as the one needing *Chamomilla*. Is flushed, restless, feverish, even delirious; may strike out or bite.

Another teething remedy is *Calcarea carbonica*, made from the oyster shell. The baby who needs *Calcarea carb.* may have a calcium deficiency, due to difficulty in assimilating calcium, and, therefore, increasing the intake of calcium doesn't help. *Calcarea carb.* promotes the assimilation of calcium.

Calcarea phosphorica has similar symptoms—delayed teething, delayed closure of fontanelles (the spaces covered by membranes where the baby's bones meet). When you choose between the two remedies, the physical makeup of your baby will be a determining factor. The *Calcarea carb.* baby is often fair and plump with a sweaty head, while the *Calcarea phos.* baby is more apt to be thin, with dark hair and eyes. How did this distinction come about? Provers who were plump and fair produced definite symptoms when testing *Calcarea carb.*, while leaner, darker persons responded to *Calcarea phos.* This sounds mysterious but it's not so strange when we consider that bodily configuration is another expression of one's individuality.

Silica, made from sand, is another useful teething remedy. The *Silica* baby has fine-textured skin, fine sandy hair, sweats about head and neck as well as feet and hands, and has an intolerance to milk. This baby is extremely bright but can be "difficult" and resents interference. I came across this *Silica* type in my own family when our grand daughter, Kathy, was in the throes of painful teething. When her older brother was miserable with the same condition, I had given him *Calcarea carb*. In a casual fashion that, I regret, is typical of "family" prescribing, I gave Kathy the same remedy, which didn't help her at all. I then realized that Kathy fit the *Silica* picture. We gave her a dose, and, within a few weeks, she brought in her first six teeth.

QUICK REFERENCE CHART

REMEDIES FOR A HAPPIER BABY

Dosage: Two tablets taken 3 or 4 times a day—or, when pain is severe, every 30 minutes to 1 hour. Decrease frequency of dosage as patient improves; discontinue when improvement is well established.

Remedy	Specific Indications	Guiding Symptoms	Worse From	Better From
Aconite For Colds	First stages of a cold Quickly settles in chest Breathing sounds harsh	Symptoms come on suddenly Onset after exposure to cold, dry winds Restlessness Anxiety; fear	Night Warm room Lying on painful side	Open air
For Croup	Hoarse, dry, croupy cough Loud, difficult breathing Grasps throat with cough			
For Diarrhea	Watery stools Crying; sleepless; restless			
For Ear infections	Swollen, hot, red, painful external ear			
For Vomiting	From nervous upset or fright Profuse sweat Increased urination			
Arsenicum album For Diarrhea	From spoiled food From too much fruit Frequent, dark, offensive stools After eating and drinking	Restlessness Weakness Thirsty for frequent small sips Burning pains	Right side After midnight Eating and drinking Cold Seashore	Heat Warm drinks
For Vomiting	From spoiled food From too much fruit After eating and drinking Nausea			
Belladonna For Colds		Sudden and violent onset Restless Red face; hot, dry skin Feverish Eyes red; sensitive to light; pupils dilated	Afternoon Lying down Touch Jar Noise	Being semierect
For Ear infections	From getting head cold or wet Generally right ear			

REMEDIES FOR A HAPPIER BABY

Remedy	Specific Indications	Guiding Symptoms	Worse From	Better From
Belladona (contd.) For Teething	Irritable Delirious: may bite or strike out	Pulse hard and pounding		
For Sore throat	Bright red			
For Vomiting	From fright From nervousness			
Bryonia For Colds	Dry, stuffy nose Dry lips Harsh, dry cough	Wants to be left alone Irritable; cries for something, then refuses it Thirsty for large drinks Constipated with hard, dry stools	Any motion or movement Touch Warmth	Rest Quiet
For Colic	Worse from movement and warmth			
For Vomiting	From fatty foods From rich foods			
Calcarea carbonica For Colic	Milk intolerance	Milk intolerance Fair, plump Sweaty head Delayed closure of fontanelles	Cold in every form Physical or mental exertion Wet weather	Lying on painful side Dry weather
For Teething	Delayed teething Calcium malabsorption			
Calcarea phosphorica For Teething	Delayed teething	Dark hair and eyes; thin Delayed closure of fontanelles	Damp, cold weather Melting snow	Summer Warm, dry weather
Calendula lotion For minor cuts and scrapes	Relieves pain Promotes healing			
Calendula ointment For diaper rash	Soothes pain Promotes healing			

REMEDIES FOR A HAPPIER BABY

Remedy	Specific Indications	Guiding Symptoms	Worse From	Better From
Chamomilla For Colic	Draws legs up Abdomen bloated	Desire to be carried One cheek red, the other pale Irritable; asks for something, then flings it aside Sleeplessness though drowsy	Night Heat Open air Anger	Being carried about Warm, wet weather
For Diarrhea	Greenish slimy stools during teething			
For Ear infections	Severe pain; wild with pain			
For Teething	Cross Sleepless though tired Greenish diarrhea			
Colocynthis For Colic	Doubles up; draws knees up Presses on abdomen	Distension of abdomen Irritable	Anger Eating or drinking even a little	Doubling up Warmth Firm pressure
For Diarrhea	Jellylike stools Severe cramping Every bite of food followed by rush of diarrhea			
Dulcamara For Diarrhea	Severe cramping Immediately following eating Green, watery, slimy, bloody, mucus stools	Onset after exposure to cold, wet weather Hypersensitive to cold	Night Cold, wet weather	External warmth Moving around
For Ear infections	Stitching pain Buzzing in ear			
Ferrum phos. For Ear infections	First stages, before ear abscesses Throbbing pain	Gradual onset Fever Pale complexion with red cheeks Restless Sleepless	Right side Touch Motion Jarring	Cold applications
Gelsemium For Colds; influenza		Lethargic Eyes droopy, heavy-lidded Fever Chills up and down back Soft and flowing pulse Thirstless Symptoms develop several days after exposure	10 A.M. Damp weather Excitement	Open air Continued motion Profuse urination

REMEDIES FOR A HAPPIER BABY

Remedy	Specific Indications	Guiding Symptoms	Worse From	Better From
Hepar sulphuris For Colds	Constant discharge Discharge yellow, from one nostril Rattling breathing Loose, rattling cough	Sensitive to draft Irritable Sweaty	Dry, cold weather	Damp weather Warmth After eating
For Ear infections	Sticking pain extending from throat to ears			
For Sore throat	Sticking pain from throat to ears			
Ipecac For vomiting	After eating Uncontrollable	Clean tongue Persistent nausea	Moist, warm wind Lying down	
Magnesia phosphorica For Earache	Severe neuralgic pain	Right side Cold Night	Warmth Pressure	
Mercurius vivus For Colds	With diarrhea	Drooling more than usual Sweaty Sick odor Weakness, trembling	Night Damp weather Sweating Lying on right side Warm room Warm bed	
For Diarrhea	Greenish, bloody, slimy stools "Never-get-done" feeling			
For Sore throat	Neck glands swollen			
Nux vomica For Colds	Nose drips daytime Nose stuffy at night and out-of-doors	Irritable Burping	4 A.M. Eating Touch	Evening Uninterrupted nap Firm pressure Damp weather
For Constipation	Strains with little result			
For Diarrhea	From overfeeding Much straining without result, or passes small amount			
Phosphorus For Vomiting	Thirst for cold water, which is vomited as soon as warm in the stomach		Evening Touch Drinking Warm food	Cold Open air Cold food Sleep
Podophyllum For Diarrhea	On bathing, eating, or drinking Forcibly expelled stool Undigested food Watery		Early morning Hot weather Dentition	

REMEDIES FOR A HAPPIER BABY

Remedy	Specific Indications	Guiding Symptoms	Worse From	Better From
Pulsatilla For Colds	For "ripe colds" Thick, creamy, bland discharge	Desires open air Wants attention Changeable	Heat After eating	Open air Motion Cold applications
For Constipation	Painful, distended abdomen	Weepy Thirstless		
For Diarrhea	From overfeeding Strains with little or no results			
For Ear infections	External ear swollen and red Thick, yellow, bland discharge; offensive odor Pain worse from heat			
Silica For Teething	Painful Delayed	Irritable; resents interference Sweats about feet, hands, head, neck Intolerance of milk Fine textured skin; fine sandy hair Alert	Morning Lying on left side Lying down Washing Cold	Warmth Wrapping up head
Varbascum For Ear infections	Generally in left ear Poor hearing	Left-sided remedy	9 A.M. to 4 P.M. Biting hard Change of temperature Talking Sneezing	

9
Your Growing Child

THE TODDLER

AN authority on babies and children describes the toddler years as "a struggle for independence and self-mastery." This is a trying time for parents, who must allow their very young children to explore their world but, at the same time, protect them from ever-present danger.

Everything a toddler gets in hand goes into the mouth, which makes parents fearful, with good reason, of a child's being poisoned or of choking. In navigating about a strange, new world, the little explorer gets a healthy share of bumps and bruises and runs the constant risk of being burned. While his body is learning resistance to disease, the small child is prone to earaches, fever, and croup. Homeopathic remedies can alleviate pain and hasten healing in many of these situations.

Poisoning

According to the U.S. National Planning Council for National Poison Prevention Week, each year 500,000 to 2 million children are victims of accidental poisoning. Ninety percent of all cases reported involve children under five years of age.

Among all drugs, aspirin is the most common cause of accidental poisoning in children. If you must use this toxic medicine, keep it out of sight and out of reach—even if it has a "safety cap." Never call baby aspirin, or any kind of medicine, "candy," and since children are natural imitators, avoid taking any kind of medicine while your child is watching. When left alone, your child may find the bottle and eat or drink its contents.

Homeopathic medicines are nontoxic; even if your child swallows the contents of an entire bottle, he will suffer no ill effects. It's important, however, to teach him that eating medicines, of any kind, is taboo; therefore, if you catch him "in the act," I recommend that you induce vomiting by tickling the back of his throat with a spoon handle. Your child will quickly associate eating medicine without permission with this unpleasant punishment.

If the medicine the youngster has ingested is toxic, call your physician.

Depending on the nature of the toxic material the child has ingested, they may advise you to give syrup of *Ipecac*, which is the only dependable means of producing enough vomiting to help in a poisoning case. For a child one year of age or older, the usual dosage is one tablespoon of syrup of *Ipecac* mixed in one cup of water. If no vomiting occurs in fifteen minutes, repeat the dose.

Even after vomiting, the child may have absorbed enough poison to produce symptoms ranging from mild discomfort to acute distress. After you follow the standard procedure just described, a group of remedies in your Home Remedy Kit can provide safe, effective means to counteract the effects of many poisons. As with all homeopathic prescribing, one must match the patient's symptoms to the symptoms of the remedy.

A British homeopath, D.M. Gibson, M.D., presents a succinct description of these homeopathic poison remedies in his book, *Homeopathy First Aid in Accidents and Ailments.*

Poisoning associated with severe vomiting and purging and extreme exhaustion with restlessness calls for *Arsenicum album.*.. With similar symptoms but cold sweat on brow and collapse, give *Veratrum album.* In marked collapse with air hunger and desire to be fanned, give *Carbo vegetabilis.* Should there be fiery burning pain on passing urine, and pallor of face, *Cantharis* is indicated. With restless tossing and great fear, a dose or two of *Aconitum* would be called for.

In addition to medicines, other common causes of accidental poisoning in children are household preparations, insect sprays, kerosene, lighter fluid, some furniture polishes, turpentine, paints, solvents, and products containing lye and acids. Some of these substances can be fatal; others, such as strong corrosives, can destroy a child's esophagus. Those potentially poisonous items that you feel you cannot do without, keep in their original containers and preferably in a high locked cabinet out of climbing reach.

BEYOND FIRST AID: If your child should swallow a strong corrosive (lye, drain cleaner, or such), or a poison containing kerosene or gasoline, *do not induce vomiting* with syrup of *Ipecac*; these substances can do more harm coming up than going down. Instead, rush the youngster to the emergency room of the nearest hospital.

Choking

Choking is the leading cause of accidental death in the home for children under age six. Candy is among the items that children most commonly choke on, but any food or nonfood is a potential killer. Familiarize yourself with the Heimilich Maneuver and subsequent homeopathic treatment (see chapter 5 on emergencies). Obtain a poster illustrating the procedure from your Department of Health, and display it in the kitchen. To prevent your toddler's choking on food:

Don't allow her to run around while eating.

Teach her not to talk or laugh with a mouth full of food.

Cut her meat in small pieces and encourage her to eat slowly.

Remove all bones from food before giving it to her.

Falls and Bruises

If your toddler is typical, he is constantly falling down, tumbling down stairs, or banging his head against a sharp table corner. Sometimes a comforting caress is enough; other times, the injury may be so severe that your child suffers shock and is sore and bruised for days.

Keep *Arnica montana* on hand for these painful mishaps. "*Arnica* should be in every house, and everybody should know of its uses," states Margaret Tyler, the renowned British homeopath. Another Britisher, Dr. Margery G. Blackie, physician to Her Majesty the Queen, agrees. "What do people do without *Arnica* in the house?" she writes. "From the time that a child begins to move about, it is prone to bruises, bumps, and minor injuries and *Arnica* can safely be called a household remedy to relieve pain, swelling, and laceration."

Another British homeopath, the late Dorothy Shepherd, who was a public health officer in blitz-torn London, recalled, "*Arnica* in potency is always given as soon as a child comes in suffering from the effects of an injury, fall, knock, cut, etc. . . It always works astoundingly quickly in reducing the swelling, relieving the pain, and shortening the period of shock and unconsciousness."

Another British homeopath, Dr. A. C. Gordon Ross, recalls that his son, aged two, fell out of his rocking chair and hit his forehead on the flagstone floor. "Almost at once a swelling appeared on the lad's forehead." His father gave him two tablets of *Arnica* and applied a cold compress of *Arnica* tincture to the swelling. "Next day the boy was as right as rain, with only a slight discoloration and tender spot to show where the injury had been."

I hear the same glowing reports about *Arnica* from patients who have small children. The other day, Dee Ann, a member of a homeopathic study group, called the office to tell me that her two-year-old had tripped on the sidewalk. "She split her upper lip; it bled for several minutes. I gave her *Arnica*, which took away the pain and calmed her, then applied *Calendula* lotion to her lip." (*Calendula* has an antiseptic and healing effect.) I've heard this kind of incident so many times I can anticipate the results: "The bleeding stopped, the bruise healed without a black and blue mark, and there was no scar."

Donald, a single parent, told me about an accident that was particularly frightening because he and his son, Tommy, live out in the country. One day five-year-old Tommy was jumping on the bed and fell into the blanket box. "He had blood all over him. His eyes were rolling back in his head, his tongue lolling out. I had no phone and my house is over a mile from the road. I gave him *Aconite* for fright, then waited five minutes and gave him *Arnica* for shock and to heal bruises and tissues." After gently washing the child's cuts with water, then applying *Callendula* lotion as an antiseptic, Donald gave him another dose of *Arnica*, and, in case there was any internal damage, continued this every half hour for three hours. A doctor examined the boy the next day, Donald said, and was impressed with the speed of healing.

Even in a severe accident that requires professional care, *Arnica* can be a tremendous help. One evening our two-year-old grandson, John Taylor, was playing in the bathroom while his mother took a bath. Anne didn't worry about his escaping from the room because he had not yet learned how to open a door. At the sound of his father's voice, John Taylor suddenly mastered the doorknob trick. He ran out, pitched headlong down the stairs, and broke his leg. Anne gave him several doses of *Arnica* fifteen minutes apart. *Arnica* can't mend a hairline fracture of the femur (thigh bone), but it helped eliminate shock, calmed the frightened child, and, later minimized swelling in the cast.

Tincture of *Arnica* is helpful, too, in relieving bruises or sprains. Rub lightly on a bruised area as you would apply rubbing alcohol. But *do not apply if skin is broken* as *Arnica* tincture will cause an irritation. When skin is broken, soak the injured part with *Calendula* lotion after cleansing with water (soap and water if wound is dirty). Then apply *Calendula* ointment to protect the injury. Repeat this process of soaking and dressing until the wound has healed. If the wound is deep, the dressing should not be disturbed for several days.

Burns

The very young and the very old are the most common victims of the 2 million burns that occur in the U.S. each year. The death rate from fires and burns is highest among persons sixty-five years or older *and among children less than five years of age.* Most burns take place in the home; roughly two thirds of fire deaths occur in residences. (See chapter 5 on emergencies for information on how to treat major and minor burns.)

According to the Shriners' Burns Institute in Cincinnati, the most common cause of burns in the U.S is hot water. Most home water heaters are set at temperatures producing water hot enough to cause a serious burn in less than five seconds. The institute recommends turning down the thermostat setting on the water heater to 125 degrees fahrenheit, which is adequate for washing dishes and clothes.

Eighty percent of the children who receive scald burns turn on the hot water, or increase its flow, while left unattended in the bathtub. To prevent scald burns from hot water, never leave a child in the bathtub for even a few seconds to answer the phone or attend to other children. If something crucial demands your attention, take the child out of the tub.

Another common cause of scald burns in young children is from boiling liquids such as water, soup, grease, and coffee. Do your best to prevent these burns by keeping your child away from the stove or table when you're pouring hot liquids. When pouring grease from skillet to can, make sure that the grease can is away from the edge of the counter. Many households use place mats rather than a tablecloth to avoid the risk of a child's tugging on the cloth, thereby overturning a receptacle containing hot coffee or tea.

Dr. Bill Gray, a homeopathic physician in Fairfax, California, told about a three-year-old he had treated for burns while working in a hospital emergency room. The little girl had upset a coffee pot, and her entire right arm and shoulder were burned raw.

"She was screaming bloody murder, which made it impossible for me to treat her," Dr. Gray said. "I put two tablets of *Cantharis* on her tongue. She calmed down immediately and went to sleep while I saw her twenty-four hours later, the skin on her arm had completely formed an outer layer. It was still pink and irritated, but it had begun to heal itself."

Causticum, a mineral preparation, is another effective internal remedy for burns. (Use whichever you have on hand.)

Dorothy Shepherd, in her book, *Homeopathy for the First-Aider*, recalls treating a boy of two who had spilled a cup of scalding tea over his right arm. "I heard his screams of pain as I rushed up the stairs to his room, his sleeves had been torn off and part of his skin with it. He would not let me touch it. The first thing I did was to give him a dose of *Causticum*; in seven minutes, as I timed it, the shrieks ceased and he allowed me to apply a dressing of *Hypericum* to the scalded area. . . . The gauze dressing was left on for a week, just moistened with the *Hypericum* when it became dry, about four or five times during the day. *Causticum* was continued every four hours. The burn... healed without sepsis in ten days without any contraction of the skin, only with the usual slight pigmentation of the skin."

As Dr. Shepherd advises, you'll need *Hypericum* tincture for external application. When a burn requires a dressing, it's important to keep the dressing moist to prevent it from sticking to the burned area. To prepare a soothing lotion with which to moisten the dressing, put one-half teaspoon of *Hypericum* tincture in one cup of clean water.

For a burn requiring a protective ointment, use *Urtica urens*, made from the stinging nettle, which can quickly relieve the burning, stinging pains that it causes. The British homeopath Margaret L. Tyler writes: "Make an infusion by pouring boiling water on stinging nettles, and cover the burn with clean linen steeped therein..." *Urtica urens* ointment is an easier way of doing this, but the homeopathic principle is the same.

Not all burn remedies come in bottles or tubes. There's one that's always fresh, sterile, decorative, and impossible to mislay. This is the *Aloe vera* plant, known for its healing properties, which should be in every kitchen. The Aloe is a succulent that belongs to the lily family; it is a perennial plant native chiefly to South Africa. Each leaf contains a jelly-like substance that soothes and heals burns. Use the bottom leaves for medicinal purposes; nick the leaf at both edges about an inch from the stalk, then break off.

If your child suffers a minor burn, do the following:

1. Give *Arnica* at once to combat shock.
2. Split the leaf of an *Aloe vera* plant in two, flatwise; scrape off the gel and apply to the burn.
3. If you don't have an *Aloe vera* plant, pour *Hypericum* lotion over the burn. Prepare from *Hypericum* tincture—one-half teaspoon to one cup of clean water.
4. Give *Cantharis* every ten to fifteen minutes if needed to relieve pain and promote healing.

Repeat whenever pain returns.

Earaches

Some children develop an earache as the aftermath to a cold; in others, an earache comes on suddenly after playing outside without a hat, or riding in a car with the window open. Try to determine the cause of your child's earache. This will help you select the right remedy. (See section on "Earaches" in chapter 8, "A Happier Baby.")

BEYOND FIRST AID: In small children, an ear infection can develop into meningitis (inflammation of the thin membranes covering the brain and the spinal cord). For this reason, physicians usually prescribe an antibiotic when a child develops an ear infection. In twenty years of practice, I have probably prescribed an antibiotic fewer than twenty times. I reserve allopathic medicines for the infrequent crisis in which I need to buy time.

If your child's earache does not respond promptly to administration of a homeopathic remedy, seek professional help at once.

Fever

This condition is alarming to new parents, but after some experience with homeopathic methods they learn to view fever not as an enemy but as a friend. An elevated body temperature is evidence that the defense mechanism is waging a battle against some invader. The fever will serve as a useful indicator of the progress of the battle if not tempered with by antifever drugs.

When your child has a fever, observe him carefully, and select the remedy whose symptom picture is most like the one he presents. (For information about remedies that are frequently indicated for feverish states, see chapter 5, on emergencies.)

Resist the temptation to give your child aspirin. Suppressing a fever opposes the body's natural efforts to heal itself. By artificially lowering body temperature, you are tampering with the indicator of your child's condition, and will have no way of knowing the true extent of the illness.

In the early 1970s, three Philadelphia pediatricians were mystified as to why a dozen children admitted to St. Christopher's Hospital for Children were bleeding from the stomach. Each child was hospitalized for several days and underwent extensive diagnostic tests that revealed no cause for the gastrointestinal hemorrhage (GIH). The doctors finally hit on the culprit—all the children had recently received aspirin "in generally accepted therapeutic doses." The link between aspirin and severe GIH in adults is well known, but these pediatricians, prior to this study, had not been aware that children suffered the same side effect. They warn parents not to give aspirin to children who exhibit any gastrointestinal symptoms such as pain or nausea.

BEYOND FIRST AID: If your child's temperature rises abnormally, say, to 105 or 106 degrees fahrenheit, contact your physician. While awaiting his or her directions, sponge your child's body with tepid water, drying each part before sponging the next.

Croup

Croup is an inflammation of the larynx (voice box), trachea (windpipe), and sometimes the bronchi (the air passages between the windpipe and the lungs). It usually strikes children two to four years old. The child starts off with a mild upper respiratory infection followed by the hoarseness that characterizes laryngitis. Then, usually at night, he wakens with a dry, barking, ringing cough.

Homeopaths have three fine croup remedies that have relieved this condition for more than 150 years—*Aconite, Spongia tosta,* and *Hepar sulphuris.* Dr. Boenninghausen, a renowned German physician born in 1843, treated croup exclusively with this trio of remedies. "Hardly one in a hundred children received all three remedies," his biographer writes, and the doctor successfully treated over 400 cases. First, give *Aconite* at the onset of croup. Here the cough is dry, loud, and barking and the child is exceedingly restless and anxious. This is the very picture of *Aconite.* If, after an hour, symptoms persist, give a second dose of *Aconite.* This is usually all that is needed.

If, however, after another hour, your child's breathing is harsh and hard and the barking, ringing cough continues, give *Spongia tosta.* This remedy is made from the toasted sponge.

At this point, your child will probably be asleep and comfortable, but, if toward morning coughing continues and breathing is still not smooth and easy, give *Hepar sulphuris*. Here the cough is loose and rattling and deeper toned.

Rarely do we need more than *Aconite* in treating croup. I give each parent of a toddler a packet containing these three remedies. If the parent calls at night reporting the beginning of croup, I advise softening a tablet of *Aconite* in one-half teaspoon of water, and giving it to the child. I ask that the parent call back if the child is not better within an hour. In such a case, I then recommend giving the second remedy, *Spongia*, in the same manner, but I seldom receive a second call.

THE SCHOOL-AGE CHILD

Attending school exposes your child not only to a succession of challenging experiences but to a host of diseases as well. So, unless you're very lucky, you can expect colds, possibly tonsillitis, and, sooner or later, one or more childhood diseases. You might not expect warts but, for some reason, they will frequently develop in older children. In addition, bed-wetting is considered a problem in this age group, and emotional difficulties may emerge. Homeopathy can help in all these varied situations.

Colds

When your child catches a cold, you can make her more comfortable and speed her recovery with a well-chosen homeopathic remedy. Study the list of cold remedies for colds in chapter 8, "A Happier Baby." Carefully observe all symptoms in order to choose the remedy that will help your child's particular type of cold.

Nutrition is one of the many factors that a homeopath considers in treating a child with recurrent colds. Rather than being concerned with a drippy nose or a sore throat, we aim to improve the functioning of the whole body, which will in turn improve the child's resistance to disease, including colds. Plenty of fruits, vegetables, and lean meats—the protective foods—rather than an excessive amount of sugars and starches constitute a proper diet. According to a naturopath, G. E. Poesnecker, director of the Clymer Health Clinic in Quakertown, Pennsylvania, "Most childhood respiratory problems stem from an improper diet, and it is only by the permanent change of his diet that a true cure can be achieved."

In your anxiety for your child's quick recovery from a cold, don't give him any drugs—prescription or nonprescription. The common cold is caused by susceptibility to virus, and no antibiotic has been found effective against viruses. Furthermore, antibiotics do nothing to improve the ability of the child's system to produce antibodies, and thus to resist disease. Nevertheless, until recently, doctors were prescribing penicillin and other antibiotics for minor infections.

One of the chief ingredients of cold and cough remedies is an antihistamine, which is useless in preventing or treating a cold and merely covers up annoying symptoms. (For a fuller discussion, see chapter 6 on colds, coughs and earaches.) Nose drops dry up nasal secretions—Nature's way of excreting germ-laden mucus. Cough syrups suppress the cough—another physiological way of eliminating poisons and clearing air passages. Most cough syrups also contain a generous helping of alcohol.

Tonsillitis

Tonsils are two small lumps of lymphatic tissue, one on each side of the throat near the base of the tongue. The adenoids, made of similar tissue, lie in the throat behind the soft palate. These tissues are situated at a point where the blood, loaded with germ-eating white corpuscles, comes closest to the surface. They act as natural traps for invading bacteria and in the process of destroying bacteria, they become enlarged and inflamed.

For an occasional attack of tonsillitis, the following remedies will ease discomfort and speed recovery:

Apis mellifica. Indicated where there is stinging pain and rosy redness of the swollen tonsils. You may see little areas on the tonsils where whitish secretions are gathering. The child isn't thirsty and has an aversion to being touched.

Baryta carbonica (barium carbonate). One of the most frequently indicated remedies. It suits mild cases that come on after slight exposure to cold or winds, and where colds tend to go into tonsillitis. The tonsils become chronically enlarged because of recurring bouts of inflammation.

Belladonna. Suits those children whose tonsillitis comes on suddenly and violently. The youngster is fine in the morning but by afternoon has a high fever and a sore throat with swollen, bright-red tonsils. As in all *Belladonna* ailments, the child is restless, without thirst although burning hot, and light hurts the eyes.

Calcarea phosphorica. Suits the child with pale, flabby-looking tonsils that are chronically enlarged. Hearing is impaired.

Ferrum phosphoricum. Helps cases in which there is smooth swelling and redness of the tonsils, a slight fever, and chronic enlargement.

Hepar sulphuris. Useful where there is a need to localize inflammation; it has sticking pains like splinters in the throat, which is extremely sensitive to touch. Pains shoot into the ears on swallowing. The child is apt to be chilly, sensitive to drafts, sweaty, and irritable.

Kali muriaticum. Helps when the throat looks gray and spotted with white. The tonsils are greatly swollen and there is much mucus.

Mercurius. Sometimes needed when there is deep redness of the whole tonsillar area. There is increased saliva and the child has very bad breath. Neck glands are apt to be swollen and tender.

BEYOND FIRST AID: The child who has frequent bouts of tonsillitis will benefit from constitutional treatment from a homeopathic physician.

Now that medicine has recognized the protective function of tonsils and adenoids, the tonsillectomy is no longer a rite of passage for children entering school. Nevertheless, nearly 1 million tonsillectomies are still performed annually, and approximately 600 youngsters die each year from hemorrhaging and other complications of the procedure.

Undoubtedly, tonsillectomy or adenoidectomy is justified where there is chronically impaired breathing or persistent loss of hearing due to blockage of the eustachian tubes. But where no urgency exists, many physicians believe that removing tonsils robs the child of part of the body's defense mechanism. We prefer to develop the child's resistance with good nutrition and constitutional treatment and avoid the trauma of surgery. If your pediatrician advises tonsillectomy and/or adenoidectomy, it may be wise to obtain a second opinion.

Childhood Diseases

With the exception of scarlet fever, which is a streptococcal (bacterial) disease, most childhood diseases are viral infections that produce antibodies specific to the infection and so usually provide lifetime immunity to those same infections. Since antibiotics do not destroy viruses, they are of no use in treating these conditions except where bacterial conditions develop, such as middle-ear infection in measles. I have rarely, if ever, seen complications in a childhood disease that has been treated homeopathically.

Measles (Seven-Day Measles). A child who contracts measles will have a fever of 102 to 104 degrees fahrenheit. Watery red eyes, sensitivity to light, and a hard, dry cough are symptoms. The child seldom has an appetite and has a coated tongue and sick-smelling breath. On the fourth or fifth day, an itchy red rash blossoms out, lasting four to seven days. The fever begins to drop when the rash appears. Natural measles (not altered by previous immunization) run for around ten days. Although measles are most contagious two to four days before the rash appears, keep your child isolated for five days after rash breaks out.

There are many homeopathic remedies for children with measles, among them the following:

Aconite. Child is restless; eyes ache in the light. Eyes and nose are streaming; there is a hard, croupy cough. This remedy is useful only in the early stages.

Belladonna. This medication fits the child who is restless, flushed, thirstless; has a sore throat and is bothered by noise, light, and jarring.

Bryonia. When the rash is slow to appear, or doesn't develop fully, *Bryonia* will bring out the rash and relieve symptoms. The cough is dry and painful and is aggravated by motion. The child is thirsty for large amounts of cold water at long intervals.

Dulcamara. This remedy is often needed when the onset of illness follows a sudden change to rainy, cold weather.

Euphrasia. Eyes are sensitive to light; tears stream from red, swollen eyes and irritate the cheeks. Watery nasal discharge does *not* irritate nose and upper lip. There is a harsh cough; child may complain of headache.

Ferrum phos. Another early stage remedy. Symptoms are similar to *Aconite.* Child is restless and anxious.

Gelsemium. Child is lethargic; doesn't want to be disturbed. Is chilly though feverish, complains of aching. Has a harsh, croupy cough, hoarseness, a watery nasal discharge that irritates the nose and upper lip. When the rash comes out, there is much itching.

Kali bichromicum. When the rash appears on fourth and fifth day, the fever usually falls and the cough will be looser in daytime. Laryngitis may develop with hoarse, brassy cough. Earache and nausea often add to discomfort. Eyes water and eyelids stick together.

Pulsatilla. Symptoms are similar to *Kali bichromicum* but milder. The cough is dry at night but looser in the daytime. Symptoms are worse at dusk.

Rubella (German Measles). Unlike measles, rubella—or German measles—is usually a mild disease. Symptoms are a low-grade fever, mild aching, and tenderness in the nodes at the back of the neck. The child may have a headache and a runny nose. The rash appears on the first or second day of the disease and lasts only one to three days.

We have a small group of remedies for rubella.

Aconite. Symptoms appear suddenly; the child has a fever, flushed face, and is restless. This remedy is seldom useful if given after the first day.

Belladonna. Symptoms are similar to *Aconite*; give after the first day or if *Aconite* did not help.

Ferrum phos. Symptoms appear gradually; fever, rosy spots in the cheeks rather than a general flush. Child is chilly with frequent sweats but wants head kept cool. Has a soft, rapid pulse and is moderately thirsty.

Pulsatilla. The child feels better in the open air. Is apt to be a little weepy, wants company and sympathy, and is irritable if not given enough attention.

A pregnant woman who has not had rubella and is exposed to a child with the disease should see a homeopathic physician. She may receive an internal prophylactic remedy, *Rubella nosode.*

Chicken Pox. Chicken pox is usually a mild disease, but occasionally a child may be very ill with it. Fever and discomfort are mild; there is a loss of appetite, and irritability. Over a period of several days, pimplelike eruptions appear on the body in successive crops. These gradually become blisters, then pustules that finally crust over. Itching can be very annoying.

The incubation period is two to three weeks after exposure, which is longer than most childhood diseases. The disease remains communicable from a few days before onset until the last lesion has crusted over.

Homeopathic remedies can help a child who has chicken pox.

Antimonium crudum. The patient is irritable and doesn't want to be touched, bathed, or even looked at. Exhibits a white-coated tongue.

Antimonium tartaricum. This patient is irritable and whining and wants company. The eruption takes the form of large pustules.

Pulsatilla. A weepy but not so irritable child who is thirstless despite the fever.

Rhus tox. Likely to be indicated when itching is extreme. Extreme mental and physical restlessness marks this patient.

Sulphur. Like *Rhux tox.*, the rash is extremely annoying. Child is very thirsty and hungry but takes more than can eat.

Mumps. This is another childhood disease that is usually mild, but can be severe in older children and adults. Symptoms are painful swelling at the jawline on one or both sides, fever, and often a headache. The simple swelling of cervical nodes is often mistaken for mumps, but if the ear lobe is pushed out, it is likely to be mumps. Isolate the child for

nine days or until glandular swelling has subsided.
You can ease the mumps patient's discomfort with a homeopathic remedy.

Apis. The swelling is soft and puffy, rosy-looking, and tender. The patient is not thirsty.

Belladonna. The patient is restless, with a red, flushed face and eyes sensitive to light. Although the skin is burning to the touch, child is thirstless.

Bryonia. Hard swelling with tenderness appears. The slightest motion, as in turning the head, is painful. The child is irritable; lips are dry and may be cracked; thirsts for large quantities of cold water.

Pulsatilla. Administer if disease lingers. The patient is weepy and whining, thirstless, and craves open air.

An adult who has not had mumps and is exposed to a child with it should take three doses of *Rhux tox.*, as a prophylactic, eight hours apart.

Scarlet Fever Scarlet fever symptoms are sore throat, chills, fever, and vomiting. The rash is a diffuse, pinkish-red flush that blanches on pressure, with noticeable whiteness around the mouth and a strawberry tongue. The rash may cover the entire body; it appears on the second day and lasts from four to ten days. The child is most contagious during the twenty-four hours before symptoms are noticed, and from two to three weeks afterwards, unless pencillin has been given.

Unlike the childhood diseases we have discussed, scarlet fever is caused by the same type of bacteria that causes strep throat and will respond to penicillin. If your child is allergic to this drug, or you wish to reserve its use for a crisis, *Belladonna*, if indicated, will shorten the course of the disease and alleviate discomfort. The majority of scarlet fever patients present the classic *Belladonna* picture, which is flushed face, fever without thirst, skin dry and burning to the touch, restlessness, not thirsty, sensitivity to light and noise. A person exposed to scarlet fever should take *Belladonna* in the prophylactic dose which is once a day for three days. Stop if unusual symptoms appear and contact a homeopathic physician.

Warts

Warts are common in older children. A wart is a growth that may be raised and hard or soft and fleshy. It appears on the hand, finger, toe, sometimes in streaks or clusters on the face. Warts are caused by a virus that enters the body through any minor break in the skin. There, it causes skin cells to grow into a small lump.

There are several homeopathic remedies that have warts as a prominent symptom. *Causticum* is for the painful wart near a fingernail or fingertip. *Dulcamara* will help the wart that is hard, smooth, and flattened. The person with a large, jagged wart who experiences stinging pains may need *Nitric acid* (potentized). The soft, fleshy wart that seems to be on a stalk is one indication for *Thuja occidentalis*, made from the arbor vitae.

Warts are related to a weakness in the person's immunological system, so it is not surprising that homeopathic treatment, which is concerned with bodily defenses, helps those troubled by these lesions. Sometimes the results are so dramatic, at least to persons new to homeopathy, that we homeopaths become known as "wart doctors"!

I got this undeserved reputation treating Peter, a twelve-year-old boy with a wart on his right index finger that was swollen and inflamed and pained him whenever he used his hand. His mother told me it had not been this sore until a doctor tried to remove it by freezing it with liquid nitrogen. At this point, Peter could not write or throw a ball. Because the wart was located near the tip of the finger and was painful, I prescribed *Causticum*. Peter's mother telephoned a few days later. The swelling had gone down and the wart was smaller. Two weeks later, the wart was entirely gone.

A patient named Jenny told me that her elder daughter, then thirteen, had plantar warts (warts on the sole of the foot). At that time, Jenny had not discovered homeopathy, and took her daughter to a dermatologist, who removed the warts surgically. They came back several months later and again were removed surgically. Recently, Jenny's younger daughter aged ten, developed a cluster of plantar warts. I recommended a dose of *Thuja*. A week later, Jenny called me. "More warts are coming out!" I told her not to worry; this was a normal action of the body, and would not continue. Three weeks later, all the warts had vanished, and there has been no recurrence in several years.

Cauterizing warts, or removing them surgically—once standard treatment—is losing favor. As dermatologist Lawton C. Gerlinger, M.D., of Centerville, Ohio, explained it, "I don't like to treat warts with surgery because scars are permanent and warts are not."

Enuresis (Bed-Wetting)

Several years ago, a television drama about a track star portrayed in flash back how he had attained his skill. At age twelve or so he had been a bed wetter. His mother, in an effort to shame him out of his habit, would hang his soiled sheets from his bedroom window. Each time he wet the bed, the boy would race home from school to remove the humiliating evidence before his friends saw it.

In this enlightened age, it's hard to imagine a mother punishing a bed wetter in such a cruel fashion. But even with the most understanding parents, a child who wets the bed endures a great deal of torment and anxiety.

The situation is frustrating for parents, too. Those who investigate the problem will find a wealth of theories and conflicting opinions concerning the cause and management of enuresis, the medical term for bed-wetting. Some authorities think that bed-wetting is caused by an organic or nervous disorder, while others blame either rigid toilet training or oversolicitous parents. But here are some generally accepted conclusions.

Enuresis is not considered a problem until the child is of school age, commonly after five years of age for girls and six for boys.

Boys are more apt to be bed wetters than girls.

There is a strong hereditary factor; in over 50 percent of cases, one or both parents were bed wetters.

Bed-wetting is rarely a sign of deep-seated psychological problems.

More often, such problems are the result of parental reaction to prolonged bed-wetting.

Scolding, shaming, or physically punishing the child rarely helps and may prolong the habit.

Homeopathy offers several remedies that, if correctly chosen, will cure many cases of bed-wetting. If your child is a persistent bed-wetter, have him or her examined by a physician to make sure there is no organic problem. Then choose the remedy that most closely matches all of the symptoms. Dosage is two tablets three times a day. Reduce frequency of dose as soon as child improves. Discontinue when improvement is established.

Belladonna will help the child who sleeps so deeply he cannot wake up. The *Belladonna* child is sensitive to jarring, as when someone bumps the bed, to change of weather or being chilled; sweating may bring on this child's bed-wetting. Incidentally, Indians of the Rocky Mountain area gave small doses of the plant nightshade, from which *Belladonna* is made, to children who wet at night.

The child who needs *Causticum* wets the bed in the first sleep and is worse in dry, clear weather. He or she has weakness and spasms in various parts of the body; urine may spurt whenever the child coughs.

Equisetum, which is made from scouring-rush, was proved in the mid-nineteenth century. Many provers reported wetting the bed. *Equisetum* often fits the child who has dreams or nightmares when urinating.

Kreosotum, made from a beechwood distillate, is often effective for the child who sleeps so deeply he or she cannot wake. The child needing *Kreosotum* may dream of urinating or has nightmares involving fire or of being pursued.

Pulsatilla will benefit the child who is shy, sensitive, weepy, and affectionate. Such a youngster is upset by sudden changes in the weather. Dr. Margery Blackie, physician to Her Majesty the Queen, says that she refers the child who wets the bed to an osteopath to adjust the lower spine, and then, where the symptoms fit, gives *Pulsatilla*. Dr. Blackie reports a high rate of success.

Sepia suits many children who wet the bed in their first sleep. This is also a symptom of *Causticum* and, consequently, it is difficult to distinguish between the two remedies. In general, the child who needs *Sepia* loves vigorous exercise and dancing, and is sensitive to cold air.

Remedies for bed-wetting, like everything else, must be chosen with the individual in mind. Some time ago, a former patient of my predecessor's came to me for treatment. After her appointment, she said, "I don't know what to do about my stepson. He wets the bed just as my daughter did. Could you give him the same remedy that the doctor gave her?" Looking up the daughter's record, I found that *Equisetum* had solved the problem, and, being pressed for time, I gave my patient several doses of the same remedy. Several weeks later, she reported that her stepson was still wetting the bed, so I asked her to bring him in. Examining the boy, I noted his characteristics—mild, gentle disposition, often on the verge of tears, loved playing out-of-doors, abhorred any kind of fat. No wonder the first remedy hadn't worked. All his symptoms pointed to *Pulsatilla*, which subsequently cured his bed-wetting.

On their doctor's advice, parents have restricted fluids after the evening meal, lifted the child at night to urinate in the bathroom, eliminated certain foods such as milk, chocolate and cole drinks. According to the author of an article in a pediatric medical journal, no specific therapy, other than reassurance and counseling, has been successful. An alarm attached to the bed or to the child that rings as soon as the youngster starts to wet is another training device, but often the child dislikes it, or members of the household object to the disturbance.

Many doctors treat bed-wetters with drugs, the most popular being imipramine hydrochloride, an antidepressant, that supposedly prevents the bladder from emptying by controlling the nerves to the bladder muscles. Whatever the action, results are doubtful. According to two pediatricians who base their findings on 2000 cases, "Children have not responded well to imipramine." The most common adverse effects of the drugs are nervousness, sleep disorder, and mild gastrointestinal disturbances. Less frequent side effects include constipation, convulsions, anxiety, emotional instability, fainting, and collapse. The *Physician's Desk Reference* warns that "overdose in any amount must be considered serious and potentially fatal."

Fears and Anxieties

Not all children's fears are deep-seated ones that require professional help. Your child may be emotionally upset by a sudden happening—a playmate moving away, the threat of a new baby in the family, a reprimand from a favorite teacher.

Sometimes sudden anger can trigger an upset stomach or other minor digestive ills in a child. One day, our granddaughter Kathy, then eight, stormed home from school. "A girl stole my pencil case!" At dinner, she ate without much appetite and later complained of a stomachache. We gave her a dose of *Nux vomica*, which "settled" her mind as well as her stomach.

If an acute emotional upset causes a child to grieve or feel anxious or fearful, *Ignatia* will help. David, aged eleven, who yearned to play on the soccer team, was crushed when he learned that he had not been chosen. When his mother told me that David had been despondent for days, I told her to give him a dose of *Ignatia*. Soon after, he forgot about his disappointment, and found that his athletic skills were better suited to track.

It is comforting to have these two self-help remedies that can relieve the youngster who experiences a sudden emotional upset. Do *not* give these acute remedies for every momentary "low" mood, but reserve them for the time when your child is overwhelmed by some event.

This is also an area in which the homeopathic physician can be of great help with constitutional prescribing. The homeopath regards the patient as an individual and does not separate the mental symptoms from the physical; all are considered as part of the total expression of the disorder and all are considered in the choice of a constitutional remedy.

BEYOND FIRST AID: If you notice any significant change in your child's behavior that recurs or persists for any length of time, this may signal a chronic emotional problem. Consult your physician.

THE ADOLESCENT

Adolescence is stressful, exciting, frustrating . . . If you're the parent of a teenager, your choice of adjective may depend on what day—or hour—you consider this. Every adolescent is different, but the bodily changes that each experiences produce similarities in behavior. Girls may welcome menstruation as a tangible sign of womanhood yet be distressed over minor symptoms. Acne is a constant worry. Mononucleosis may bring school and social life to a halt, and emotional problems frequently appear during adolescence.

Some of these matters require the services of a homeopathic physician. Other situation you can handle yourself, with a carefully chosen homeopathic remedy and a good dash of commonsense.

Menstruation

Most girls have minimal discomfort during their periods—a dull headache, a low, nagging backache, cramps the first day or two. Many experience a down-in-the-dumps feeling a few days before and on the first day of the period. Some of the discomfort comes from physiological changes—muscular contractions of the uterus and changes in the secretion of hormones—but attitude toward menstruation has a lot to do with it. A gynecologist once said, "If a mother has experienced painful menses, so will the daughter."

So, when you discuss menstruation with your daughter, emphasize that it is a normal, healthy function. If, now and then, she complains of pain, the simplest way to relieve discomfort is by giving the correctly chosen homeopathic remedy The keynote for *Magnesia phosphorica* is "relieved by warmth," often the case with menstrual cramps. In such a case, dissolve ten tablets of *Magnesia phos*. in one cup of hot water, sip every few minutes during period of cramping. Acute, severe pain of this type responds more readily to the repeated dose.

Occasionally, a girl will double up and press a pillow or book into her abdomen to relieve cramps. She will probably be relieved by *Colocynthis*, which has in its provings the symptom "relieved by hard pressure." *Colocynthis* is also indicated for burning pain in the ovarian region and restlessness.

One time my daugher Della was miserable with menstrual pain. I tried to help her but she was impatient and snappish. I suddenly realized—she's asking for *Chamomilla*. This is a remedy for a child or adult who is ornery and "impossible" while in pain. After Della received one dose of *Chamomilla*, the pain disappeared and so did her bad temper.

Belladonna is the remedy for bearing-down pain that feels as if the uterus is trying to come out. Pain comes and goes suddenly, and the person expels bright red blood. A young houseguest of mine once had severe cramps. When she said, "I feel as if everything is coming out," I knew she needed *Belladonna*. This remedy brought her prompt relief.

Apis, a remedy we associate with insect bites, relieves the person who experiences stinging pain in the ovarian region. Symptoms are: violent bearing-down pains as if the person is in labor; scanty, dark, bloody mucus; and scanty dark urine.

Pulsatilla is one of the prime remedies for delayed or suppressed menses, provided that the young woman is not pregnant. I once gave *Pulsatilla* to a teenager who complained of a missed period but insisted she could not be pregnant. The following month, when her period failed to return, I ordered a lab test and, yes, she was pregnant. At a time like this, I am grateful that a homeopathic remedy, even when not called for, does not cause serious side effects.

COMMONSENSE MEASURES: Place a heating pad or hot-water bottle on the abdomen. Yoga exercises can help relieve menstrual discomfort. Diaphragmatic breathing, which is used in preparation for childbirth, is good for relieving muscular stress of any kind. Other exercises are the "child's pose," "cat stretch," and a half-shoulder stand, which takes pressure off the uterus.

In addition to a well-balanced diet, one or more of the following supplements and vitamins may help:

Brewer's yeast is a generally good supplement. Start with one-half teaspoon per day, gradually increase to two to three tablespoons per day. Too much yeast at first may cause discomfort due to excessive intestinal gas formation.

Vitamin E protects tissues and apparently reduces the oxygen requirement. Take 800 units once a day, starting three days before the expected period.

Calcium lactate or bone meal helps in painful muscular conditions; one bone meal capsule contains phosphorus, which is essential for normal skeletal growth and maintenance. Take six tablets of whichever you have on hand.

Kelp, a sea plant with high iodine content, helps the thyroid. Low thyroid states often seem to be accompanied by menstrual difficulties. Take at least three tablets of kelp each day throughout the month.

BEYOND FIRST AID: If severe pain persists despite self-help measures, physiological difficulties—a retroflexed uterus (bent backwards), adhesions, or a congenital defect—may be the cause. If so, surgery may be required. Your homeopathic physician will be able to facilitate postoperative recovery by means of a series of carefully selected remedies.

Acne

Many teenagers experience some form of acne. This is an inflammation of the sebaceous (oil) glands that are found just beneath the surface of the skin, especially that of the face, upper back, and chest. At puberty, when glandular activity increases, the sebaceous glands enlarge and begin to secrete a greater amount of a skin lubricant called sebum. If the gland canals become clogged, the sebum accumulates and the glands swell until they rupture. According to some authorities, the sebum becomes irritating to the surrounding skin, and a pimple results. This is the beginning of inflammatory acne.

Before we talk about what homeopathy can do for acne, let me explain how the homeopath feels about treating skin ailments in general. A skin ailment often is a sign that the body's defense mechanism is working. Homeopaths have observed that ailments progress from the outside to the inside, from less important organs to more important organs, as a disease deepens. Conversely, cures proceed from within outward; the disorder recedes by transferring itself from a more important organ to a less important organ. We therefore get rid of ailments in the reverse order from that in which they developed. For example, a patient recovering from hepatitis called me to tell me that she had developed a skin rash on her thighs. "What should I do?" "Don't do anything," I said. "This shows we're on the right track!" The process of cure was following the reverse pattern of the disease process, that is, moving from within outward, from liver to skin, which is the proper direction of homeopathic cure. So we don't always want to interfere with a skin problem.

Acne, however, can benefit from homeopathic treatment. A constitutional remedy usually helps acne, but if I can't determine this, sometime I give *Kali bromatum*, which is known to be helpful in treating acne. If, in addition to itchy acne, your teenager is restless during sleep and has unpleasant dreams, these are further indications for *Kali brom*. *Sulphur* is a good remedy for the teenager with chronic acne characterized by a rough, hard skin that gets worse from washing. This same person is often warm blooded, perspires freely, and suffers from constipation. *Antimonium tartaricum* has often cleared obstinate cases of acne in which there is much formation of pustules. *Hepar sulphuris* will abort painful boils that develop pus, or quickly bring them to a head.

COMMONSENSE MEASURES

1. Clean the face with a soft complexion brush or a hard-knit Vic, a cotton washcloth made in England. Use pure castile soap (no medicated soaps); rinse well. Pat on witch hazel for mild astringent effect.
2. Eliminate chocolate, soda pop, salted nuts, and other oily foods. Avoid processed foods, TV dinners, packaged snacks, and all food with chemical additives and preservatives.
3. Take zinc gluconate 30 mg. per day. Many patients have reported considerable improvement after starting this supplement.

Current medical opinion is that diet does not affect acne. In a recent magazine article, Dr. Sidney Hurwitz, a clinical professor at Yale University School of Medicine, says that he was wrong in telling acne patients to stay away from chocolate and potato chips.

Gustave H. Hoehn, M. D., author of *Acne Can Be Cured*, does not agree. "Diet is the answer to the acne problem," Hoehn says. The common ingredient found in the native diets of Italians, Koreans, Japanese, and Eskimos is thin oils—olive oils, fish oils, peanut and vegetable oils—while we Americans eat heavier fats, which are found in milk, cheese, and ice cream as well as in bacon, ham and pork, and lard used in many fried foods. He points out that Italians, in their native country, have beautiful complexions, as do Koreans, Japanese, and Eskimos. But when these people move to the United States, their descendants develop acne like other Americans.

Paavo Airola also, in his book *How to Get Well*, stresses the relation of diet to adolescent acne. "Avoid animal proteins, including milk . . . animal fats . . . all sweets, chocolate . . . soft drinks, candies, ice cream and everything made with sugar and white flour.

I've had many patients with acne, and I am convinced that a proper diet is essential for a good complexion. Many a teenager's acne has improved by merely eliminating milk and chocolate.

Girls face the same problems as boys, except that it is socially approved for them to cover skin blemishes with makeup. Recently Phyllis, a young research chemist in cosmetics, said, "I wouldn't use any of the stuff I work with." Phyllis feels as we homeopaths do: Work with the body rather than against it. If the skin is dry, find out the reason, rather than smearing on cream. If the skin is oily, it requires more than applying witch hazel. *Secrets of Beauty through Health*, by Edgar Cayce, provides information on do-it yourself skin aids and cosmetics that can supplement the adolescent girl's dietary efforts.

Cautionary Notes. For a girl with severe acne, dermatologists sometimes prescribe an oral contraceptive pill, which contains the female hormone estrogen and tends to limit the production of sebum. This action interferes with the hormonal balance of the body, a risky and suppressive interference. Side effects from the pill range from nausea, vomiting, and weight gain to persistent headaches, depression, impaired liver function, and blood clotting. This seems a high price for a girl to pay for an improved complexion.

For both moderate and severe acne, the standard treatment is oral antibiotics. According to Drs. W.J. Cunliffe and J.A. Cotterill, authors of *The Acnes*, the "drug of choice" is tetracycline. If this drug doesn't work, the authors recommend three other antibiotics, one of which is clindamycin. If the patient still doesn't respond, the authors suggest a "three-pronged" attack, namely, an oral antibiotic along with topical treatment and x-ray therapy.

If a dermatologist recommends antibiotic therapy for your teenager, consider the side effects. Symptoms such as stomach pain, vomiting, and diarrhea are more common with tetracycline, according to the writers cited above, than most other orally administered antibiotics. If the patient is a girl, a more disturbing side effect, in view of the high incidence of teenage pregnancies, is that tetracycline can permanently stain the teeth of unborn children and even interfere with enamel formation.

Clindamycin can cause ulcerative colitis. I learned this firsthand from a patient, a young woman named Lee, who had a constant sore throat. Lee, a busy executive, became impatient with homeopathic treatment, and consulted a throat specialist who prescribed clindamycin. Her sore throat improved slightly, but in the process she developed colitis, which, among other disagreeable symptoms, causes frequent, bloody stools. Severe colitis can be fatal. Lee and I worked months to overcome the consequences of the antibiotic.

Chloramphenicol, another antibiotic used for acne, has produced depressed bone marrow in a significant number of cases. The bone marrow is no longer able to produce the white blood cells needed to fight infection, and overwhelming infection can result.

Acne can be very disturbing for a teenager, but no amount of mental anguish can justify using drugs with such potential for harm. If an antibiotic can affect the teeth of the unborn, its action is more than skin deep. The medical literature contains a case study of a sixteen-year-old girl who developed a malignant growth while receiving long-term tetracycline therapy for acne. This is a rare occurrence but one that cannot be dismissed.

In general, homeopaths are wary of treating skin ailments per se. If we have acne and apply an ointment, or take an oral antibiotic, we have suppressed the disorder, and the disease progresses inward. It seems more than coincidence that a great many persons with asthma, in their youth had eczema that was treated with suppressive ointments. In this case, the disease went from the outside inward, from a less important area, the skin, to a more important part, the respiratory system.

Improved diet and hygienic skin care, along with either a homeopathic constitutional remedy or acute remedy, will alleviate the acne without endangering the adolescent's health.

Mononucleosis

Mononucleosis, or "mono"—also known as the "kissing disease"—is common among young people. Symptoms are a grippelike malaise, chilliness, fatigue, and headache, followed by high fever, sore throat, swelling of lymph glands. Almost any organ can be affected.

Mononucleosis is an infection of the lymph system that lasts from two weeks to two months. The disease is communicable from just before symptoms appear until fever and sore throat are gone. To prevent infecting others, the patient should dispose of tissues and wash hands after coughing or blowing nose, as with a cold.

A homeopathic remedy, *Cistus canadensis* (Canadian rock rose), is frequently indicated in mono cases. Andy, a college student who has been my patient since he was a youngster, recently benefited from this, but not before he had gone through some misery from allopathic drugs. Here's Andy's experience as he relates it: He had a bad sore throat, went to the student medical center, and was given ampicillin, an antibiotic. He broke out in an itchy rash all over his body. His feet became so swollen that he couldn't put bedroom slippers on and had trouble walking even to the bathroom. He went back to the doctor, who gave him benadryl, an antihistaminic, to relieve the itching. By this time, Andy had developed flulike symptoms that the doctor diagnosed as mono, and, consequently, gave him prednisone, a steroid. At this point, Andy had the good judgment to call a halt on drugs and check with me by phone.

I sent him a homeopathic preparation of ampicillin to use as an antidote, to be followed three days later by a dose of *Cistus*. Because of the well-demonstrated fact that "what a drug causes it can, in appropriate dosage, cure," we know that homeopathically prepared ampicillin can stimulate the defense mechanism to throw off the residual effect of the antibiotic, and thus help the system to overcome the drug-imposed ailments.

I also restricted his diet. Since the liver can become involved in mono, there is no use burdening it with heavy food. "Don't eat anything until you're really hungry," I said, "then start off with yogurt and fruit." Some days later, Andy reported that the rash and swelling were gradually subsiding and that he felt fine.

If the mono patient experiences abdominal fullness and discomfort, the spleen may be enlarged. Consult your doctor, who will probably advise eliminating exercise to prevent complications of the liver or spleen.

Emotions

It is not desirable for an adolescent to take medicine, even a homeopathic one, for every emotional upset. Sometimes, however, the adolescent overreacts to a setback such as the breakup of a romance or defeat in a school election; the young person grieves longer than seems warranted or experiences intense shame or some other negative emotion. At these times, it is comforting to be able to provide a homeopathic remedy to relieve the distress rather than resort to standard drugs, tranquilizers, or antidepressants that deaden the feelings and cause unpleasant side effects. The correctly chosen homeopathic remedy will enable the teenager to regain a sense of proportion.

A patient was concerned about her seventeen-year-old-daughter. The young woman had broken up with her boyfriend a month earlier and had been despondent ever since. "She's out of sorts all the time," her mother said. "She sighs continually—nothing pleases her." I suggested she give her a dose of *Ignatia*.

James Tyler Kent, whose *Repertory* is a "must" for every homeopath, describes *Ignatia* as "helpful for the suffering that results from misplaced affections or anger." This proved to be the case with this young woman. A week later, her mother called and told me that the girl had "snapped out of it." "I don't know what I ever saw in him," she said to her mother.

Pulsatilla is another remedy that is frequently recommended for young women. Kent describes the *Pulsatilla* patient as tearful, nervous, fidgety, changeable, easily led and easily persuaded, and craving sympathy; she is chilly yet feels better in the open air and can't stand a warm room.

This description fit my fourteen-year-old patient Marcella, who had not yet started her periods, and had become extremely moody in recent months. She had many *Pulsatilla* characteristics, including a loathing for fatty foods and warm rooms and a very affectionate disposition. I gave her *Pulsatilla* and, when she returned three months later, she seemed a different girl; she was pleasant and vivacious and related happily that her periods had begun.

The mother of a fifteen-year-old boy was concerned about her son's outbursts of anger. "He put his fist through another wall," she said. The boy came to see me, ostensibly about a bad knee, and I spent an hour with him learning his symptoms. Except for athletics, he was doing poorly in school. He craved sugar and starches, which gave him frequent stomaches, a bad taste in his mouth upon awakening, and constipation. His uncontrollable anger was his greatest problem. The most innocent remark could send him into a rage. Sometimes he was so angry he cried, which embarrassed him and made him even more angry.

I gave him *Nux vomica* in high potency, and a week later his mother reported that he had "calmed down." If your teenager is experiencing ill effects from anger, *Nux* in low potency will help.

Another patient, a sixteen-year-old boy named Bob, had been brooding and unhappy for weeks after losing a class election. "He thinks the election was rigged," his mother said. "He's not sleeping well, his appetite is off. He's so proud," she continued. "He won't admit he's hurt, and hates to have anyone sympathize." I told her to give him a dose of *Natrum muriaticum*, a remedy that often displays these personality traits. Some time later, when Bob's mother came in for a routine checkup, I asked her if Bob had recovered from his disappointment. "Oh yes," she said, "soon after I gave him the remedy, he forgot about the whole thing."

BEYOND FIRST AID: An adolescent with a serious emotional problem is not likely to respond to a self-help homeopathic remedy. In such a case, seek professional help.

QUICK REFERENCE CHART
REMEDIES FOR YOUR GROWING CHILD

Dosage: Two tablets taken 3 or 4 times a day—or, when pain is severe, every 30 minutes to 1 hour. Decrease frequency of dosage as patient improves; discontinue when improvement is well established.

Remedy	Specific Indications	Guiding Symptoms	Worse From	Better From
Aconite For Croup	First stages of croup Cough dry, hoarse, and barking Loud difficult breathing Hoarseness and laryngitis	Anxiety Fear, fright Fever Eyes watery, sensitive to light Restlessness	Evening and night After midnight Warm room Rising from bed	Open air
For Seven-day measles				
For Three-day measles	Useful on first day; seldom effective later			
Aloe vera plant For Burns	Pain To promote healing			
Antimonium crudum For Chicken pox		Fretful Irritable Aversion to bathing Aversion to being looked at Aversion to touch White-coated tongue	Evening Cold bathing Heat	Open air During rest
Antimonium tartaricum For Acne	Formation of pustules	Desires company Drowsy Irritable	Evening Damp, cold weather	Sitting up
For Chicken pox	Large pustules	Sweaty Whining	All sour foods Milk Warmth	
Apis For Menstrual disorders	Stinging pain in ovarian region Violent bearing-down pain as if in labor Scanty, dark, bloody mucus Menses late, with throbbing headache Soreness	Thirstless Aversion to being touched Scanty, dark urine	Right side Late afternoon After sleeping Heat Pressure Closed and heated room Touch	Cold bathing Open air Uncovering Cold applications
For Mumps	Swelling: soft, rosy, puffy, and tender			
For Tonsillitis	Stinging Pain Rosy redness of swollen tonsils Ulcers on tonsils, with whitish secretions			

REMEDIES FOR YOUR GROWING CHILD

Remedy	Specific Indications	Guiding Symptoms	Worse From	Better From
Arnica For Injuries	Pain Bleeding caused by injury Bruising injuries to soft tissues Injuries from blows, falls, or blunt objects Lacerations, cuts Shock and trauma of injury		Light touch Rest Heat	Keeping head low
Arnica lotion*	Pain and swelling of bruises, sprains, strains			
Baryta carbonica For Tonsillitis	Onset after slight exposure to cold or winds Mild cases Tonsillitis from almost every cold Stitching and smarting pain when swallowing; worse with empty swallowing Tonsils chronically enlarged because of recurring inflammation	Takes cold easily Bashful	Lying on painful side Thinking of symptoms Washing	Walking in open air
Belladonna For Bedwetting	Sleeps so deeply, cannot wake up	Thirstless Restless Drowsiness with inability to sleep Sensitive to light and noise Skin flushed and hot to the touch	Afternoon Touch Motion Noise Jarring Light Lying down	Sitting up Standing
For Seven-day measles				
For Three-day measles	To follow *Aconite* if not improved			
For Menstrual disorders	Menses bright red Menses too early Menses too profuse Bearing-down pain as if uterus trying to come out Pain comes and goes suddenly			

*Externally for massage or as a compress, only if skin is unbroken.

REMEDIES FOR YOUR GROWING CHILD

Remedy	Specific Indications	Guiding Symptoms	Worse From	Better From
Belladonna (contd.) For Mumps				
For Scarlet fever	Shortens the disease and alleviates discomfort when symptoms fit. As a prophylactic when exposed			
For Tonsillitis	Sudden and violent onset. Swollen, bright-red tonsils. Throat feels constricted. Sensation of lump in throat			
Bryonia For Seven-day measles	Rash does not appear, or comes and goes. Instead of rash, bronchitis or pneumonia may develop	Cough dry and hard with tearing pain. Drowsy. Bursting, splitting headache. Irritability. Mouth dry, lips cracked. Muscle twitching. Thirsty for large amounts of cold water	Warmth. Any motion. Morning. Eating. Exertion. Touch	Pressure. Rest. Cold things. Lying on painful side
For Mumps	Hard swelling with tenderness			
Calcarea phosphorica For Tonsillitis	Tonsils pale and flabby. Tonsils chronically enlarged. Hearing impaired	Cold extremities. Feeble digestion	Damp, cold weather. Mental exertion	Summer. Warm, dry weather
Calendula lotion* For Injury	Applied externally to broken skin to: Cleanse, Aid healing, Control bleeding, Relieve pain			
Cantharis For Burns	Pain. Rawness and smarting. To prevent infection	Raw, burning pains	Approach. Touch	Cold applications

*One-half teaspoon succus to one cup water.

REMEDIES FOR YOUR GROWING CHILD

Remedy	Specific Indications	Guiding Symptoms	Worse From	Better From
Causticum For Bed-wetting	During first sleep at night From slightest excitement Urine spurts when patient coughs, sneezes	Muscular weakness Restless at night	Dry, clear weather Cold draft Becoming cold Getting wet	Damp, wet weather Head of bed Warmth
For Burns	Pain Ill effects of burns Old burns that do not heal well			
For Warts	Near fingernail or fingertip On nose Large and jagged Painful Bleed easily			
Chamomilla For Adolescent moods	Impatient, whining restlessness Snappish	Thirsty Hot Night sweats	Night Heat Anger Warm applications	Warm, wet weather
For Menstrual disorders	Irritable Pain unendurable Profuse discharge of clotted, dark blood			
Cistus canadensis For Mononucleosis	Sore throat Swollen, painful glands	Extremely sensitive to cold	Slightest exposure to cold air Mental exertion Excitement	Eating
Colocynthis For Menstrual disorders	Bearing-down cramping Boring, burning pain in ovary Doubles up from pain Great restlessness	Irritable	Anger Indignation	Hard pressure Doubling up Warmth
Dulcamara For Seven-day measles	Less nasal discharge and aching than *Gelsemium*	Aversion to food Burning thirst for cold drinks Fever with chilliness and thirst Onset after sudden change to rainy, cold weather	Night Cold Damp, rainy weather	External warmth Moving about
For Warts	On face On palms of hands Smooth and flattened			

REMEDIES FOR YOUR GROWING CHILD

Remedy	Specific Indications	Guiding Symptoms	Worse From	Better From
Equisetum For Bed-wetting	Dreams or nightmares when urinating From habit, no other cause	Frequent urging to urinate Sharp, burning pain while urinating	Right side Movement Pressure Touch Sitting down	Afternoon Lying down
Euphrasia For Seven-day measles	First stages of measles Eye symptoms very pronounced	Cough dry and harsh Eyes: Bright, red, swollen, sensitive to light, streaming tears irritating to cheeks, burning and swelling of lids Headache intense and throbbing Watery nasal discharge that does not irritate nose and upper lip	Evening Indoors Warmth Light	Dark
Ferrum phos. For Three-day measles	Fever begins to drop after appearance of rash	Anxiety Fever with chilliness Frequent sweats Headache helped by cold applications Moderate thirst Pulse soft and rapid Restless "Roses" in cheeks	Night 4 to 6 A.M. Touch Jarring Motion Right side	Cold applications
For Seven-day measles	Fever begins to drop after appearance of rash			
For Tonsillitis	Smooth swelling and redness of tonsils Chronic enlargement			
Gelsemium For Seven day measles	Itching increases when rash appears	Chilly Aching Cough harsh and croupy Doesn't want to be disturbed Fever Hoarseness Lethargic No thirst Watery discharge that irritates nose and upper lip	Damp weather Motion Tobacco smoking Any effort to think Anticipation	Open air Increased urination
Hepar sulphuris For Acne	Painful boils filled with pus Prickly pain	Helps localize infection Chilly Sensitive to drafts	Before midnight Morning Cold drinks	Damp weather Wrapping head up Warmth

REMEDIES FOR YOUR GROWING CHILD

Remedy	Specific Indications	Guiding Symptoms	Worse From	Better From
Hepar sulphuris For Croup	After *Aconite* and *Spongia* Loose, rattling, croaking cough Suffocative, choking, coughing spells Difficult breathing with wheezing Hoarseness	Sweaty Irritable	Lying on painful side Dry, cold winds Slightest draft Touch	After eating
For Tonsillitis	Sticking, splinterlike pain in the throat Pains shoot to ears on swallowing Throat sensitive to touch			
Hypericum* For Burns	Pain To promote healing		Cold Touch Least motion	Bending head backward
For Injury	To parts rich in nerves Puncture wounds from nails, bites, splinters Smashed fingers, toes, nails			
Ignatia For Adolescent moods	Changeable Bad effects of grief, worry, shock, disappointment, anger "Lovelorn" syndrome Sad, tearful Silent brooding Much sighing	Cannot bear tobacco	Night Heat Anger Coffee Smoking	Warm, wet weather While eating
Kali bichromicum For Seven-day measles	Symptoms more intense after taking *Pulsatilla*	Harsh, dry, croupy cough Thick, yellow ropy discharges from eyes, ears, nose, throat	Morning Hot weather Undressing	Heat
Kali bromatum For Acne	Itching eruptions Worse on face, chest, shoulders	Restless during sleep Unpleasant dreams		Being occupied mentally or physically

*Lotion: one-half teaspoon *Hypericum* tincture to one cup water.

REMEDIES FOR YOUR GROWING CHILD

Remedy	Specific Indications	Guiding Symptoms	Worse From	Better From
Kali muriaticum For Tonsillitis	Throat appears gray, spotted with white Much swelling of tonsils; difficulty in breathing Much mucus		Rich foods Fats Motion	
Kreosotum For Bed-wetting	Dreams of urinating Sleeps so deeply cannot wake up Must hurry when desire comes to urinate	Anxious dreams of fire, pursuit, etc.	Cold Open air Lying down	Motion Warmth Warm diet
Magnesia phosphorica For Menstrual disorders	Cramping Menses too early Menses dark and stringy		Right side Night Cold Touch	Warmth Bending double Pressure
Mercurius For Tonsillitis	Deep redness of tonsillar area Stitching pains passed to ears on swallowing; fluids return through nose Neck glands swollen and tender	Bad odor from mouth Increased salivation Thirst for cold drinks Profuse sweating without relief	Lying on right side Night Wet, damp weather Perspiring Warm room Warm bed	
Natrum muriaticum For adolescent moods	Depressed Irritable Bids for sympathy and consolation, but irritated by it Oversensitive Ill effects of fright, grief, anger Wants to be alone to cry Sleepless from grief	Coldness Craving for salt Great weakness and weariness	About 10 A.M. Heat Consolation Noise Lying down Warm room	Open air Cold bathing
Nitric acid, potentized For Warts	Bleed on washing Large, jagged Stinging, splinter-like pains	Irritable Sticking pains appear and disappear quickly	Cold climate Hot weather	Riding in a car

REMEDIES FOR YOUR GROWING CHILD

Remedy	Specific Indications	Guiding Symptoms	Worse From	Better From
Nux vomica For Adolescent moods	Irritable Impatient Hypersensitive to noise, touch, light, odors, etc. Ill effects of anger, loss of sleep, or mental strain	Time passes too slowly Affected greatly by least ailment	Morning Mental exertion Touch Stimulants, narcotics Cold Open air Dry weather	Evening Uninterrupted nap Damp, wet weather Warmth Lying down
For Emotional upsets	Irritable Faultfinding Sullen			
Phosphorus For Emotional upsets	Fearful: of dark, death, thunderstorms, etc Depression Excitable, produces heat all over	Oversensitivity to touch, light, sound, odors, thunderstorms Sweats at night Thirst for very cold water	Evening Physical or mental exertion Thunderstorms	Open air Sleep
Pulsatilla For Adolescent moods	Changeable Given to extremes of pleasure and pain Easily led and persuaded Desires attention and sympathy Nervous, fidgety Sensitive and tearful Timid	Affectionate Nausea Chilly Thirstless despite fever and dry mouth Earache Eyes, water, stick together	Toward evening Feet hanging down After eating Heat Warm room Rich, fatty food Sudden changes in weather	Cold applications Motion Open air
For Bed-wetting				
For Chicken pox				
Pulsatilla For Three-day measles	Rash appears; Cough loosens in daytime; fever goes down			
For Seven-day measles	Rash appears on 4th or 5th day: Cough loosens in daytime; fever goes down			
For Menstrual disorders	Delayed or suppressed menses Flow starts and stops Painful, scanty flow Thick, dark, clotted menses Downward pressure Chilliness Nausea			
For Mumps	To clear up later stages			

REMEDIES FOR YOUR GROWING CHILD

Remedy	Specific Indications	Guiding Symptoms	Worse From	Better From
Rhus tox For Chicken pox	Intense itching	Restless both physically and mentally	Cold During sleep or rest	Motion Warm applications
For Mumps	Dark-red swelling Left side more apt to be affected Prophylactic when exposed			
Sepia For Bed-wetting	Wets bed in first sleep	Loves vigorous exercise and dancing Sensitive to cold air Indifferent to those loved best Irritable Sad	After sweat Cold air Before thunderstorm	Exercise Pressure Drawing limbs up
Spongia For Croup	After *Aconite* Cough dry and barking, like a saw driven through a board Wheezing, whistling, rasping Harsh, loud breathing Wakes out of sleep with sense of suffocation, loud violent cough, great alarm and difficult breathing Throat sensitive to touch	Anxiety, fright Cold patient	Before midnight Heat Talking Reading Swallowing Lying down Cold drinks	Eating or drinking warm things
Sulphur For Acne	Rough, hard, scaly skin Itching, burning	Constipated Hungry but eats little Very thirsty Burning heat, especially soles of feet	Washing Scratching Time to time Rest Bathing Warmth	Lying on right side Dry, warm weather
For Chicken pox	Intense itching			
Thuja For Warts	Soft, fleshy warts Seem to be on a stalk		Heat of bed Cold, damp air Vaccination	Left side
Urtica urens (Ointment) For Burns	To protect Pain		Water Cool, moist air Touch	

10
What Homeopathy Can Do for Women

FROM the Victorian era until recently, the American woman had abdicated control over her body. Led to believe that childbirth is analogous to a surgical procedure, she allowed herself to be sedated during labor without questioning the effect of anesthesia on her baby or herself. After childbirth, she took medication to dry up her breast milk, and during menopause, massive doses of estrogen—following doctor's orders.

This passivity isn't natural to women. As Barbara Ehrenreich and Deirdre English, the authors of *Witches, Midwives and Nurses*, point out, women have always been healers... nurses and counsellors, pharmacists, midwives, doctors without degrees, the wise women of the village." The pioneer woman in American history typifies this active role. One such woman was Hannah Livsey Harris, widowed shortly after she and her family settled in the lonely prairie of central Kansas in the 1870s. As Edward Harris, one of Mrs. Harris's four sons, describes his mother in a family journal:

> Mother had been taking care of some sick folks before coming out here and had had some experience doctoring with homeopathic medicine, which an old doctor in Marshall Country had been teaching her. He had taught her the method of preparing the medicine and had given her a doctor's book with full instructions. He told her she would probably need it when she came out west as there would be few doctors in this section, which prophecy proved to be entirely correct.
> She was soon being called out to doctor various ailments and to usher babies into the world, often riding several miles on horseback. She was especially successful in relieving the ailments of children. She was kept busy in those early days as the nearest doctor was fifteen or twenty miles away...

Happily, women are once again taking responsibility for their own health, and learning how homeopathy can help them take better care of themselves and their families.

YOUR HEADACHE: FAST AND SAFE RELIEF

According to June Biermann and Barbara Toohey, authors of *The Woman's Holistic*

Headache Relief Book, 85 percent of the 45 million chronic headache sufferers in the United States are women. We don't have any statistics on the sex ratio of those suffering from an *acute* headache but, judging by my practice, women clearly outnumber men.

Homeopathy can help most headaches. Prescribing for a headache isn't easy because there are so many different kinds of headaches, each with its own symptoms. But the results are well worth the effort.

These are the most frequently indicated remedies for an acute headache:

Aconitum nappellus. Characterized by a sudden, violent headache all around the head like a band, or in the forehead like a bursting pain. The patient is restless, fearful, and thirsty. The symptoms are worse in the evening or night, in a warm room, and on getting up from bed, and better in the open air. Such a condition often follows exposure to cold wind.

Arnica montana. Suits the headache brought on by a blow or a fall and is characterized by a sore, bruised feeling anywhere in the head.

Belladonna. A natural for the headache that comes on suddenly and violently, like the *Aconite* headache, but in addition is characterized by throbbing, pounding pain, restlessness, a hot head, and a red, flushed face.

Bryonia. One of the most commonly indicated remedies for acute headache. The pain is stitching or tearing and is most apt to be right-sided. The person feels worse from motion, even moving the eyes or raising the head. There may be a bursting sensation on stooping or on coughing. Constipation often accompanies this headache.

Gelsemium. May be needed by the person who has a vague but distressing headache beginning in the neck and extending up over the head, settling in a band around the head. It may develop into a bursting sensation in the eyes and forehead, and the scalp feels tender. It sometimes comes on after exposure to too much sun or from mental stress, bed news, or apprehension. It is worse from lying down. The *Gelsemium* patient is languid, chilly, and without thirst and wishes most to be left alone.

Iris versicolor. Often needed when a migraine-like headache begins with blurring of vision. The scalp may feel tight and there is profuse flow of saliva with burning of the tongue, throat, and stomach. The person may lose his or her appetite and there may be nausea and vomiting. *Iris* headaches are usually worse in the evening and at night, and better from continued motion.

Kali bichromicum (potassium bichromate). Matches the symptoms often referred to as "sinus headache": pain is in the "mask" area, either over, under, or behind the eyes, or at the root of the nose in a small spot that can be pointed to with one finger. Motion aggravates the pain, as does stooping or bending forward. The person feels worse from warmth, better in the open air.

Nux vomica. Has a well-deserved reputation as "the hangover headache" remedy. It is a splitting headache all over the head, with nausea and an out-of-sorts feeling. The person is irritable, oversensitive to everything.

Sanguinaria canadensis. Very often fits the typical "sick headache." It begins in the morning, increases during the day, and lasts until evening. Pain is bursting, beginning in the back of the head, spreading upward and settling over the right eye; it is accompanied by nausea and often by vomiting and dizziness.

Aspirin for Headache : Asking for Trouble

Ridding oneself of headaches can't be achieved overnight. In the meantime, if you develop a headache, please don't "take two aspirin," as many doctors and, of course, manufacturers of aspirin, who spend $100 million a year in advertising, have been urging us to do. A Drug Review Board in the U.S. investigating aspirin and an aspirin substitute, concluded that the public has been inadequately warned about the shortcomings and side effects of these products. Just because aspirin is sold as casually as chewing gum doesn't mean it is safe to take.

Aspirin can cause asthma, skin eruptions, anaphylactic shock that can result in asphyxia, and other allergic reactions. More widespread is damage to the gastrointestinal tract. As described in the September 1977 issue of *Science Digest*, "Even the usual two-tablet dose can cause unpleasant side effects, including vague feeling of stomach upset, heartburn, nausea, vomiting and, in rare instances, massive gastrointestinal hemorrhaging." According to the September 1966 issue of *Consumer Bulletin*, excessive use of aspirin may cause severe iron deficiency anemia, or damage to the bone marrow, vitally important in maintaining the composition of the blood. As reported in *Consumer Research*, aspirin can be critically dangerous for peptic ulcer patients.

Acetaminophen, an aspirin substitute, was given the same safety rating as aspirin, with one difference: Whereas aspirin overdoses produce such obvious distress that lifesaving measures can be initiated at an early stage, the symptoms of Acetaminophen overdose may not be apparent until after irreversible liver damage has occurred.

PREGNANCY

Pregnancy is a test of woman's health. If her state of vitality is high, she blooms at this time. On the other hand, if her defense mechanism is weak, pregnancy will accentuate her chronic problems.

As we have learned from tragic experience, a pregnant woman must not take any standard medical drugs, especially during the first trimester or close to the time of delivery. According to Dr. Kenneth R. Niswande, a professor of obstetrics at the University of California, Davis, School of Medicine, "Most pharmacologic agents do cross the placenta with ease, usually by passive diffusion." Evidence of the danger of drugs in pregnancy is the ruling by the U.S. Food and Drug Administration that, beginning in 1980, all prescription drugs must include all available information concerning their potential for causing birth defects.

Homeopathic remedies carry no such risk. A potentized remedy contains very little substance, and therefore, does not act directly upon organs or tissue. There is no danger of side effects. The well-chosen homeopathic remedy stimulates the body's defense mechanism, or vital force, and consequently produces an overall improvement.

Morning Sickness

Some women experience nausea and vomiting during the early months of pregnancy. Fortunately, we have a number of homeopathic remedies to alleviate this condition safely.

If even the thought of food makes you feel nauseated, think of *Colchicum autumnale*.

This is made from the meadow saffron. *Colchicum* is best known as a remedy for gout, but when indicated, is also useful for digestive upsets.

If you are thirsty for cold water, but vomit it as soon as it gets warm in your stomach, consider *Phosphorus*. If this is your remedy, one dose usually eliminates the vomiting.

Some women start the day off retching ("dry heaves") and are miserable and cranky until afternoon. Next day, the process repeats itself. If this describes your condition, you may need *Nux vomica*. *Anacardium* is similar to *Nux vomica* but has an unusual symptom. The patient retches every morning, feeling better as soon as she eats something.

If you have nausea without any of the other symptoms, try *Natrum phosphoricum* (sodium phosphate), which often relieves nausea.

Here's a home remedy to use in conjunction with a homeopathic remedy. Combine one-half teaspoon salt and one-half teaspoon honey in one pint of water. Take one teaspoon every fifteen minutes four times, then two teaspoons every fifteen minutes four times, then three teaspoons every fifteen minutes four times. This maintains a degree of hydration by sending down such small amounts of liquid that, as one patient said, "The stomach doesn't seem to notice!"

BEYOND FIRST AID: If morning sickness persists to such a degree that it interferes with your food intake, seek professional help.

Varicose Veins

During pregnancy, pressure on the veins of the pelvis from the enlarging uterus blocks the upward flow of blood from the legs, which cause veins in leg and thigh to become dilated. The most severe case I've seen was a once-again-pregnant mother of nine children whose leg veins were crooked and bulging. I told her to take two tablets of *Hamamelis* three times a day and apply *Hamamelis* tincture to the areas of inflammation. The remedy relieved the discomfort and the angry areas cooled down.

If you're suffering from varicose veins, *Hamamelis*, in both internal and external form, will relieve the pain. In addition, walk more to stimulate circulation in the legs. Elevate your legs when sitting or lying down. When you are going to be on your feet for any length of time, wear elastic stockings; put them on before you get out of bed.

BEYOND FIRST AID: If self-help measures fail to alleviate discomfort, ask your doctor about surgery.

Urinary Problems

A patient, expecting her second baby, told me she knew she was pregnant when, on several occasions, she "just made it" to the bathroom. A frequent need to urinate is common in early and late pregnancy. This is caused by the enlarging uterus exerting pressure on the bladder.

Cystitis, a bladder infection, isn't serious but is uncomfortable: you feel the urge to urinate every few minutes, but pass only a few drops, which are accompanied by a burning, painful sensation. Begin drinking eight to ten glasses of water a day, discontinue all citrus fruits, and consider the following homeopathic remedies:

Aconite. Sudden retention of urine from chill or fright.

Cantharis. Persistent and violent urging, passing a few drops at a time; may be accompanied by aching in small of back.

Mercurius corrosivus (mercury chloride). Persistent urging with intense burning, unfulfilled need to urinate, with constant urging and straining. Urine may be mixed with a little blood.

Nux vomica. Frequent and painful urging with little result.

If cystitis develops when you are away from home without your remedies, drink a generous amount of cranberry juice, preferably without sugar, and parsley tea made from the fresh or dried herb.

BEYOND FIRST AID: A severe reduction in or lack of urination is a danger signal that may indicate that the normal path of urine through the kidneys is being blocked. This condition, called pyelitis, is an inflammation of the kidney passages. Symptoms include low back pain, chills and fever, a burning sensation on urination, and sometimes swelling of the legs. To determine whether the pain of kidney origin, place hands on your hips and dig in your thumbs; if the kidney is inflamed, this will probably hurt. A kidney infection is always serious. Seek medical attention at once.

While waiting for the doctor, a well-selected homeopathic remedy will stimulate your defense mechanism to fight the infection. If you're experiencing chills and fever, swelling, and scanty urination, *Apis* is the remedy of choice. If you have deep flank pains at your waist level, consider *Berberis*, made from the prickly hedge barberry.

Constipation

Even though your bowel action is normally regular, you may experience a change in bowel function owing to the enlarged uterus pressing against the lower intestine. It's important to correct constipation since you are eliminating waste material "for two." See chapter 7 for advice on relieving constipation.

Do not take a laxative during pregnancy. You don't know how much of the laxative substance will be absorbed into your blood stream, or its long-range effect. Remember, anything ingested may cross the placental barrier, and this may affect your unborn child.

Hemorrhoids

A hemorrhoid may be caused by the fetus crowding against the lower region of the bowels. If you're troubled by this painful condition, see the discussion in chapter 7 that describes homeopathic remedies, both internal and external.

Indigestion

In late pregnancy, as your stomach assumes a more horizontal position, you may experience a burning sensation in your chest, accompanied by belching. Consider the homeopathic remedies to relieve indigestion and the commonsense measures to prevent indigestion in chapter 8.

Insomnia

Early in pregnancy, you probably felt as if you couldn't get enough sleep. In later months, with your added girth, it's hard to find a comfortable position in bed.

Dependence on any medicine, homeopathic or otherwise, is undesirable, but if you occasionally have trouble getting to sleep at night, you can safely take a homeopathic remedy that has no direct effect on the body. *Nux vomica*, known as "the student's remedy," is helpful when you're sleepless after mental strain; you can't turn off your mind. Consider *Arsenicum* when you're sleepless from anxiety or worry. *Cocculus*, made from Indian cockle, a climbing shrub, is known as "the nurse's remedy"—when you can't get back to sleep after your late night duty is done. Remember *Cocculus* when you get up to feed the baby and can't go back to sleep.

When you're sleepless from excitement or joy, *Coffea* will help. Coffea, in large doses, stimulates mental processes; the similar, in potency, will have the reverse effect. However, if you're a habitual coffee drinker, *Coffea*, for some unexplained reason, may be less effective. *Gelsemium* is difficult to distinguish from *Coffea* because both may be indicated by sleeplessness from excitement. *Gelsemium* has an element of dread or anticipation, while with *Coffea*, the mind is racing in high gear. *Pulsatilla* is like a broken record—the person is sleepless from recurring thoughts.

In view of the thalidomide tragedy in the 1960s, in which a sedative drug caused birth defects, it is difficult to imagine a woman risking her unborn baby's health by taking any kind of sleeping pill or tranquilizer. At this writing, methapyrilene, an antihistamine, the chief ingredient in over-the-counter sleeping aids, has been declared a carcinogen, so perhaps by the time you read this, these products won't be around. As for prescription sleeping pills, a 1979 report from the National Academy of Sciences in the U.S. states that these drugs are not as free of hazards as many physicians believe. For example, the report says that benzodiazepines, which are considered safer than barbiturates, tend to leave active substances in the patient's blood for a substantial period of time. If the patient is pregnant, the drug will get to the baby.

LABOR

Childbirth is a natural process and unless complications develop, no intervention is needed. More and more couples accept this view and choose labor without anesthesia and, more prefer to have their baby born at home.

Homeopathy can facilitate childbirth with the use of a homeopathic remedy to help prevent lengthy and painful labor. The early settlers learned about this remedy from the Indians, who called it "squaw-root" or "birth-root." Indian women chewed the root when they were at full term. The early homeopaths, ever on the alert for curative medicines, potentized this remedy, which they called *Caulophyllum thalictroides*.

In the event of false labor pains (pains not accompanied by effacement and dilatation of the cervix), the remedy stimulates the onset and continuation of effective contractions.

A British homeopath, Dr. Douglas M. Borland, author of *Homeopathy for Mother and Infant*, recommends taking a daily dose during the last two or three weeks of pregnancy to ease labor. In several cases, I have given *Caulophyllum* daily during the last week before the expected date, and these mothers have reported a rapid, "easy" labor.

Patricia, a fourth-generation homeopathic patient in Miami, Florida, told me about the experience of her daughter, Jan, with *Caulophyllum*. "I took her to the hospital," Pat said. The nurse examined her and advised me to go home—'It's going to be hours.' Instead, I gave Jan a dose of *Caulophyllum* and waited around the hospital. Within a half hour, she went into active labor, and the baby was born an hour later."

If you have experienced unmedicated childbirth, you know that giving birth is aptly called "labor." I was conscious of this, being persent at my daughter Anne's first delivery, a home birth presided over by another physician. It seemed as cozy as a tea party compared with the impersonal hospital deliveries to which I was accustomed. Anne worked hard and felt sore and bruised afterwards. I gave her *Arnica montana* immediately after delivery and repeated the dose every fifteen minutes until she felt comfortable. In addition to relieving sore muscles and bruised parts, *Arnica* will speedily heal an episiotomy.

Carbo vegetabilis, known as the "great reviver," proved a boon during Anne's second delivery. After labor had been going on for some time, she seemed completely and too tired to carry on. The air conditioner was going full tilt—she had asked to have it on even though the rest of us were freezing. I suddenly realized Anne needed *Carbo veg.*—besides exhaustion, its keynote is a craving for moving, cold air. I gave her a dose, and, in minutes, she had her strength back to complete the job.

In a hospital setting, the induction of labor is sometimes accomplished by rupturing the membranes enclosing the infant or by giving the mother a medicine that stimulates the uterus to contract. According to Emanuel A. Friedman, M. D., Professor of Obstetrics and Gynecology, Harvard Medical School, "The practice of elective initiation or augmentation of labor *without clearly defined indication* has become increasingly popular in recent years... Induction of labor is not completely devoid of hazard."

POSTPARTUM BLUES

Baby blues sometimes hit mothers on the third day after birth; others feel sad and weepy for a longer period. Few experience true postpartum depression, which requires psychiatric help. What causes the blues? A shift in hormones occurs after childbirth, coinciding with a "let-down" feeling after the high of pregnancy and delivery. A new mother often feels unable to cope with her new responsibility, which compounds the problem.

In most cases, the blues will disappear by themselves, but if you're experiencing this, it's a shame to suffer at this time when the correct homeopathic remedy can help you change your mood.

The woman who has been irritable since giving birth may benefit from *Kali carbonicum*. She is tired and weak, unlike her usual self, and sensitive to every change in weather.

Betty, a patient I've treated during two pregnancies, had regained her energy very quickly both times after having her babies. This last pregnancy was different. Although she had good reason to be tired with two small children and a new baby, on her last visit, she seemed not only fatigued but depressed. Betty is fair complexioned, of a stocky build, and tends to put on weight easily. Her eyelids often seem a little puffy. She dislikes cold weather and tires easily. In addition, she worries a great deal and doesn't like to be alone. All these symptoms fit *Kali carb.*, a remedy known to be helpful in ailments following childbirth. Shortly after taking a dose of *Kali carb.*, Betty reported that she felt more energetic and the gloom had lifted. She wondered what had made her so low in spirits, and was overjoyed to be her old self again.

If you feel weepy and sigh a great deal, consider *Ignatia*, known as the "sighing remedy." If your sadness seems more deep seated, *Natrum muriaticum* is a better choice. The *Natrum mur.* patient wants to be alone, weeps at the slightest provocation, but tries to conceal her feelings. She is worse when consoled. She either craves salt or has an aversion to it.

BREAST-FEEDING

A breast-fed infant has fewer infections, better digestion, and is healthier in later life than a bottle-fed baby. So, if possible, nurse your baby. All infant formulas are inadequate attempts to duplicate mother's milk, and none is as good as the original.

If breast-feeding is not a tradition in your family, you may be concerned about producing enough milk to satisfy your baby.

Richard Moskowiz, M. D., of Santa Fe, New Mexico, a family doctor who is in favor of home births or "rooming-in," believes that every mother will be able to breast-feed successfully if she suckles her baby early enough. Here's what Dr. Moskowitz advises: "The best way to promote the milk flow is to encourage the baby to nurse *immediately* after cutting the cord, and to have him/her continue to nurse as often as possible during the first few days until the milk supply comes in."

If Dr. Moskowitz's advice comes too late for you to follow, or, if despite diet and enough rest, your milk supply is not adequate, homeopathy offers two useful self help remedies. If you suspect that your problem is from emotional strain, I suggest that you take *Ignatia amara*, two tablets three times a day. *Ignatia* is a wonderful remedy for the effects of mental stress connected with shock, bereavement, disappointment, or distress.

If emotional stress is not a strong factor, take *Calcarea phosphorica* in the same dosage. *Calcarea phos.* is made from phosphate of lime, which is essential to the proper growth and nutrition of the body. Within a few days, you should notice an improvement in milk supply.

Women under homeopathic constitutional treatment don't usually have this problem, but for many others, the remedies mentioned above have turned a frustrating breastfeeding experience into a happy one.

BEYOND FIRST AID: Difficulty in producing milk may be symptomatic of a larger problem, and the best way to treat this is through homeopathic constitutional treatment. The constitutional remedy, prescribed by a physician, will strengthen a woman's entire system and, in so doing, increase her milk supply.

After the milk flow is established, you may notice a tender reddened area on the breast or near the nipple, which most likely indicates a plugged milk duct, known as "caked breast." This plugged milk duct is generally caused by inadequate emptying of the breast, and will soon be relieved by frequent nursing. If the soreness is accompanied by fever, and sometimes chills and aching, it is most likely a breast infection. In my experience, the best cure for a breast infection is a hungry baby and a dose of *Phytolacca decandra*. This remedy, made from poke root, cures the majority of breast infections, and I've seen it work countless times.

At time of birth, breasts quickly become engorged, swollen with blood, and tender.

Sometimes when the breast is full, the baby clamps down with hard little gums on the nipple, which becomes irritated, then cracks and bleeds. To keep nipples soft, rinse off the baby's saliva after each feeding, and apply olive oil or vitamin E oil. Toughen tender nipples by exposing them to the air. Drop the trapdoor in your nursing bra and leave it open as much as possible. The plastic lining in the bra holds in moisture and keeps out air. To prevent this, keep a sterile pad in each cup and change it frequently when it becomes moist.

Do not let anyone, family member or doctor, induce you to stop nursing because of a breast infection or a bad cold or flu. Probably the only valid reason to discontinue nursing is tuberculosis. A contagion is not transmitted to the baby through the milk; if you're concerned about your baby catching your germs, wear a mask.

MENOPAUSE

A time of despair... fear of madness... no longer a real woman... This was how menopause was depicted in our Western culture until this last century. According to Wendy Cooper, an English journalist, this attitude stemmed from the belief that menstruation was a form of purging in which women were relieved of evil humors and toxic substances. Menopause, the cessation of menstruation, meant that these evil humors were being retained within the body.

Menopause, stripped of superstition, is a period of transition when the ovaries stop producing eggs and the uterus ceases its periodic changes and resultant bleeding. Most women today regard it as a natural and inevitable development and suffer no ill effects. Perhaps 20 percent experience mild symptoms, and a small percentage some nervous symptoms and mild disorders.

Your reaction to menopause, like any other periods of your life, will depend mainly on your state of health. The person whose vitality is low may have problems with bleeding, hot flashes, headaches, and fatigue. One's degree of serenity is also a factor. The high-strung woman may encounter some emotional problems or be troubled with insomnia.

BEYOND FIRST AID: All of these menopausal symptoms can be helped by homeopathic constitutional treatment. This is the process by which a homeopathic physician selects and administers a woman's own constitutional remedy based on the totality of her symptoms. This is the best way I know to strengthen the body's vital defenses and restore a healthy balance and sense of well-being. It is not a question of treating a woman's ovaries or her psyche; her entire being needs help. Menopause is not an acute illness and, except in the case of insomnia, does not lend itself to self-help remedies.

The Estrogen Question

If you are troubled by any of the symptoms of menopause, you may have considered taking estrogen, the female sex hormone administered to women whose own natural supply of this hormone is waning. According to one psychiatrist, estrogen therapy in the menopausal patient produces a feeling of normal well-being and improves the entire emotional state of the patient.

Not everyone agrees that estrogen is beneficial. As reported in the *FDA Drug Bulletin*, "New research affirms that menopausal and postmenopausal women who take estrogens have an increased risk of endometrial (uterine) cancer. The only established way to use estrogens with minimum risks in women with intact uteri is to prescribe low doses for relatively short periods—i.e., months, rather than years."

Unless you are going to take estrogen for the rest of your life, sooner or later you must experience the shifting of the hormone balance, and some of the symptoms that accompany this change. Our own defense mechanism is well equipped to make the necessary adjustments without the interference of a drug whose purpose is to block the normal action of the body. Taking estrogen is a risky and expensive way of postponing the inevitable readjustment that Nature has decreed.

QUICK REFERENCE CHART
WOMEN'S PROBLEMS

Dosage: Two tablets, taken 3 or 4 times a day—or, when pain is severe, every 30 minutes to 1 hour. Decrease frequency of dosage as patient improves. Discontinue when improvement is well established.

If you are under the care of a homeopathic physician, *do not take any remedies for acute illness without checking with your doctor.*

Remedy	Specific Indications	General Symptoms	Worse From	Better From
Aconite For Headaches	Heavy, hot, bursting, throbbing headache Sensation as if band around head Fullness in forehead	Sudden, voilent onset Restless Fearful	Lying on painful side Night Warm room Cold, dry winds Tobacco smoke Music	Open air
For Urinary problems	Cystitis Sudden retention of urine from chill or fright Painful urination Scanty, red, hot urine Anxiety on beginning to urinate			
Anacardium For Nausea of pregnancy	Retching in morning Morning nausea relieved by eating Empty feeling in stomach, always nibbling	Impaired memory	Hot application	Lying on side Gentle massage
Apis For Urinary problems	Burning and soreness when urinating Scanty urination	Chills Fever Swelling Thirstless	Right side Touch Pressure Heat	Uncovering Open air Cold bath
Arnica For Childbirth	Sore muscles following childbirth Bruised parts and bruised feeling Promotes healing of episiotomy	Sore, lame feeling Bruising to soft tissues	Least touch Rest Damp cold weather Wine	Lying down Keeping head low
For Headaches	Onset after blow or fall Sore, bruised feeling anywhere in head			
Arsenicum For Insomnia	From anxiety or worry Restlessness Wants head raised by pillows	Irritable Thirst for small drinks often Desires air but sensitive to the cold	After midnight Wet weather Cold Cold food or drink	Heat Having head elevated Warm drinks

WOMEN'S PROBLEMS

Remedy	Specific Indications	General Symptoms	Worse From	Better From
Belladonna For Headache	Throbbing pain Eyes red; pupils dilated; sensitive to light Face flushed Head hot	Sudden onset Restless Thirstless	Least exertion Lying down Slightest noise Even slight jar	Firm pressure Sitting up Tightly wrapping head
Berberis For Urinary problems	Burning pains Pains deep inside kidneys extending into bladder Sensation as if some urine remaining after urinating Backache	Rapidly changing symptoms	Motion Standing Any sudden jarring movement	
Bryonia For Headaches	Apt to be a right-sided headache Head feels as if it would burst Sharp, stitching, tearing pain Pain from slightest cough Thirsty, but drinking makes headache worse (from motion of swallowing)	Irritable Dryness of lips, tongue, lining of nose Constipation	Coughing Drinking Least motion Sitting up Stooping	Lying on painful side (because it prevents motion) Rest
Calcarea phos. For Breast-feeding	Deficient breast milk	Colic pains whenever she eats	Mental exertion	Warm dry weather
Cantharis For Urinary problems	Cystitis Persistent and violent urging Passing few drops at a time Aching in small of back Cutting and burning pains	Unquenchable thirst with aversion to all fluids	Touch Urinating Drinking cold water or coffee	Gentle massage
Carbo veg For Childbirth	Exhaustion during labor, "too weak to finish the job"	Desire for moving air Sweat cold and clammy	Lying down Wine Coffee Milk	Fanning Cold Belching
Caulophyllum For Childbirth	False labor To stimulate the beginning and continuation of effective contractions	Erratic pain and stiffness in small joints (fingers, toes, etc.)		

WOMEN'S PROBLEMS

Remedy	Specific Indications	General Symptoms	Worse From	Better From
Cocculus For Insomnia	Unable to get back to sleep after late-night work is done Constant drowsiness	Motion-sickness Weakness during menstruation	Loss of sleep Emotional disturbance Menstrual period Open air Eating Smoking	
Coffea For Insomnia	From mental activity, excitement, joy Sleeps until 3 A.M., then only dozes	Intolerance of pain Nervous agitation	Excessive emotions Narcotics Noise Strong odors Open air	Warmth Lying down
Colchicum For Insomnia	Smell of food causes nausea Craving for various things, averse to them when smelling them Aversion to food, drink, tobacco	Great weakness Internal coldness Thirst	Loss of sleep Mental exertion Smell of food in evening Any motion	Stooping
Gelsemium For Headaches	Onset after exposure to heat of sun, mental stress, bad news, apprehension Bursting sensation in eyes and forehead Pain begins in neck, extends over top of head Tightness; sensation of band around the head	Wants to be alone and quiet Does not want to be moved Chilly Thirstless	Emotion Any effort to think Tobacco smoking Thinking of one's ailments	Profuse urination Stimulants
For Insomnia	Scalp sore to the touch From excitement about a coming event, tobacco, exhaustion Cannot get fully asleep			
Hamamelis For Varicose veins (Tablets internally; lotion externally)	Bruised soreness of affected parts	Bleeding, sore hemorrhoids		Warm moist air

WOMEN'S PROBLEMS

Remedy	Specific Indications	General Symptoms	Worse From	Better From
Ignatia For Insomnia For Post-partum blues (Check diet!)	Jerking of limbs on going to sleep Long, troubling dreams Weepy Frequent sighing Changeable mood	Bad effects of grief, disappointment, worry, shock Sensitive, excitable patients	Morning Emotions Strong odors Tobacco smoke Open air	Change of position While eating Hard pressure Walking
Iris versicolor For Headaches	Migraine or sick headaches beginning with a blur before eyes Scalp feels tight, especially right temple Nausea and vomiting	Burning of tongue, throat, and stomach Profuse flow of saliva Loss of appetite	Evening Night Rest	Continued motion
Kali bichromicum For Headaches	"Sinus headache" symptoms: pain in the "mask" area or at the root of the nose Vision blurred Blindness; vision returns as headache increases Desires darkness; quiet; to lie down Bones and scalp feel sore	Tough, stringy discharges which adhere to parts Nose stuffy and crusty; bleeds when crusts are removed	Morning Motion, walking Stooping Bending forward Hot weather	Pressure Warm food or drink Fresh air
Kali carbonicum For Post-partum blues (Check diet!)	Irritable since giving birth Unlike usual self Aversion to being alone Tiredness	Weakness Backache Sensitive to every change in weather	3 A.M.	Daytime Moving about
Mercurius corrosivus For Urinary problems	Cystitis Persistent urging with intense burning Constant urging and straining, need to go and can't Urine may have small amount of blood Perspiration after urinating		Evening Night Acids	At rest
Natrum phosphoricum For Nausea of pregnancy	Nausea Sour eructations and vomiting	Excess of acidity		

WOMEN'S PROBLEMS

Remedy	Specific Indications	General Symptoms	Worse From	Better From
Nux vomica For Headache	Often helpful in "the hang-over headache" from over-indulgence in rich food and drink Dizziness, nausea and sour vomiting Splitting headache, in back of head or over eyes, as if nail driven in Frontal pain with desire to press head against something Scalp sore to touch Headache in the sunshine Headache associated with stomach problems	Oversensitive to light, noise, music, everything Irritable, especially in morning Chilly, sensitive to drafts	Morning Mental exertion After eating Touch Spices Stimulants Narcotics Cold	Evening Uninterrupted nap At rest
For Insomnia	After mental strain Cannot sleep after 3 A.M. until toward morning, awakes feeling wretched			
For Nausea of pregnancy	Begins day with retching, "dry heaves" Nausea in morning, after eating Weight and pain in stomach			
For Urinary problems	Cystitis Frequent and painful urging with little result			
Phosphorus For Nausea of pregnancy	Great thirst for cold water, which is vomited as soon as it becomes warm in the stomach Weak, empty, gone feeling in abdomen	Fearful, anxious Sudden onset of symptoms Very sensitive to outside impressions: light, noise, thunderstorms, odors, etc.	Evening Touch Physical or mental exertion Warm food or drink	Sleep Cold Cold food Open air
Phytolacca decandra For Breast-feeding	"Caked breast" (plugged milk duct) Breast hard and very sensitive During nursing, pain goes from nipple all over body	Restless Fever Chills Aching, sore feeling	Right side Night Motion	Warmth Rest

WOMEN'S PROBLEMS

Remedy	Specific Indications	General Symptoms	Worse From	Better From
Pulsatilla For Breast-feeding	To dry up mother's milk when no longer needed	Sensitive, weepy Desires attention and sympathy Changeable symptoms Thirstless Desires open air	Heat Warm room Rich, fat food	Open air Cold food and drink
For Insomnia	From recurring thought Wide-awake in evening			
Sanguinaria For Headache	Burning in eyes Bursting pain; begins in back of head in the morning, increases during day, lasts until evening; spreads upwards; settles over right eye Headache from sun "Sick-headache"; with chills, nausea, vomiting, dizziness Periodic headache; may return every seven days or at time of menses	Burning sensation in various parts of the body Red burning cheeks	Lying on right side Motion Touch Sweets	Darkness Lying down Quiet Sleep Acids

11

Keeping Your Pets Healthy

THE other day Eleanor, a patient I've treated for several years, called. After a few minutes of pleasant conversation, I asked, Any flareup of your arthritis? No, all was well with her. After a pause, she said, "I hate to bother you but we're so concerned about Freddy, our Yorkshire terrier. He's having seizures and the vet can't do anything for him."

I assured her that I didn't mind having Freddy as a patient. Animals of all varieties including barnyard animals, canaries, pigeons, a pet mink (to mention some that I've heard about) benefit from the well-chosen homeopathic remedies just as humans do. It's particularly gratifying to treat an animal homeopathically because no one can claim that the remedy has merely a placebo effect—"it's all in your mind."

In this chapter, we will share some of our animal experiences and others related by a dog breeder and goat owner, among others.

To get back to Freddy, Eleanor related that the Yorkie had all the signs of an epileptic seizure—during an attack he would fall on his side, clamp his jaws, and foam at the mouth. Consulting my *Materia Medica*, I selected *Calcarea phos.*, which has these symptoms, and recommended that she give a tablet three times a day. A month later, Eleanor wrote that Freddy had not had another seizure, and seemed better in general.

Dr. Wilbur Bond, a homeopathic physician, discovered that homeopathy worked for animals when his dog, a cross between a Pomeranian and a miniature coolie, caught a bad chest cold. As Dr. Bond had a neighbor who was a veterinarian, he consulted the vet, who prescribed penicillin. Being disinclined to use antibiotics except in a critical situation, Dr. Bond wrote in an article, "I decided to try my hand at prescribing." He noted the dog's physical symptoms—hoarseness, sore throat; and mental symptoms—afraid of thunderstorms, has a jolly disposition. Then, using the time-honored method of repertorizing the principal symptoms of a case, Dr. Bond gave his pet a dose of *Phosphorus*. The dog soon revived. "He went hopping along with a little spring in his step . . . and the cold disappeared from his lungs like magic."

Some conditions respond to specific remedies, which makes prescribing an easy matter. A dog with vomiting and diarrhea or any stomach upset frequently needs *Arsenicum alb*. This advice was related by Barbara, a patient who breeds Shi-tzus, those dogs with straight white hair that look like walking mops. If *Arsenicum alb.* fails to relieve symptoms, Barbara gives *Veratrum alb.*—three doses eight hours apart.

Aconite is another remedy that this dog breeder uses frequently—for a dog with a scratched eye, and for those with beginning colds and coughs as well. *Aconite* has the mental symptom of fright that Barbara recently discovered applies to dogs, too. "A bitch just had a litter—she was so frightened after the experience she wouldn't touch her puppies. I gave her *Aconite*—there was a complete personality change." Barbara routinely gives *Arnica* to the mother after delivery, and sometimes later, *Pulsatilla* "to help clean up the uterus."

Ruth Holland, trustee of the American Foundation for Homeopathy and animal lover, told us how to care for a pugnacious dog who comes home with cuts and bruises. "Wash his wounds with *Calendula* lotion, then if he's bleeding, give him *Phosphorus* or *Ferrum phos*. If the wound is inflamed, give *Hepar sulf.* to localize the infection.

"Animals have emotions just like people," Ruth continued. Her mother's dog, a terrier, was inconsolable after her mistress' death. "I prescribed *Ignatia* for her grief," Ruth said, "and she soon perked up." Ruth gives *Ignatia* to her own dog when he comes home out of sorts from a kennel stay.

We've always had cats, both alley and pedigreed, so I've treated a great many feline hurts and ailments. The worst injury I can remember happened to a scrappy tomcat who came home one day with all the skin and some of the flesh removed from his neck—you could actually see the trachea and the jugular vein. Although I feared the end was near, I prepared *Calendula* lotion (ten drops of the succus to a cup of lukewarm water), then dipped sterile balls of cotton in the lukewarm lotion and sponged the open wound. I continued sponging twice a day, or whenever I could snatch a few minutes. No pus developed and the wound healed nicely; after some weeks, to my surprise, the fur grew back.

Tommy, another battle-scarred veteran, came home from a fight with his forearm badly swollen and oozing pus. I put *Hepar sulf.*, which tends to localize an inflammation, in his milk. The infection subsided but the wound failed to close. So, I gave him *Silica*, having found this remedy to be a good treatment for wounds that heal slowly, and that completed the job.

Ear canker in a cat, which often interferes with balance or creates an abscess in the middle ear, is helped by *Hepar sulf*. This we learned from Ms. Raymonde Hawkins, principal of an animal rescue center in Sussex, England. This experienced prescriber has treated her charges homeopathically for many years.

Relating by mail her varied experiences (that include restoring a parrot's plumage with the help of *Selenium*), Ms. Hawkins reported success in treating "cat flu," a form of gastroenteritis with watery diarrhea, with *Arsenicum alb.*: one dose three times a day for three days.

Since horses usually represent a large investment, let's hope the owner of one reads the following incident. Recently, Christine, an experienced homeopathic prescriber, witnessed a freak accident at a riding stable. A high-strung horse, unnerved by some disturbance, reared up, fell over backwards, and, in the process, bit his tongue, severing a major artery.

As Christine recalled, "He was bleeding like a fire hydrant. I told the stable boy to get some ice and I ran to the car for my kit of remedies that I keep in the glove compartment. Meanwhile, someone had called the vet, who said there was nothing he could do—he couldn't patch a tongue. I gave the horse one dose of *Phosphorus*, which soon stopped the bleeding." Christine subsequently learned the horse's tongue had healed satisfactorily.

Our authority on goats and homeopathy is Evelyn Purser, who has a goat farm in

Sacramento, California. As coauthor Jane learned during a visit with Evelyn, this friendly, energetic, gray-haired lady has treated her goats homeopathically for several years; she's so enthusiastic about the results that she's giving a study course in the subject to her goat-raising neighbors.

Evelyn's students raise such questions as: "My new doe stumbled off the milking stand. She's crippled, her front leg is bothering her, she doesn't want to walk. What should I do?" Evelyn reads from a basic text, which advises: Give two *Arnica* tablets every half hour until she shows improvement. If stiffness remains, follow up with *Ruta*.

Next class session, the student who had asked the question reported that, after one dose of *Arnica*, "I saw the goat stretch and move a little. After four doses, she was walking." Evelyn also gives *Arnica* to the doe that is exhausted by prolonged labor, or to a goat in shock. She keeps *Arnica* within reach for "when I wham my shinbone against the milking stand."

Prescribing for an animal, as for a person, requires careful observing. Knowing whether your dog is chilly or warm, for example, is important in choosing a remedy. To determine this, observe whether he curls up in a warm place to conserve body heat or stretches out in a doorway to catch the breeze. Does he like very cold drinking water? Yes, if he likes you to run water in a sink instead of drinking from his bowl. How about his preference for fats, another important symptom? Next time you toss him a bone, notice if he carefully eats around the fat.

A pet's mental symptoms are easy for an owner to determine. You know better than anyone whether your pet is friendly and agreeable, or the reverse. When your pet is ailing, note any deviations from normal behavior. Has he lost his appetite? Instead of bounding over to greet you, does he barely raise an ear? Is she asking to be let out more frequently or straining when using her cat box? As every parent knows, you don't need verbal communication to size up a patient's condition.

Although I enjoy conversing with my patients about their pets, and mine, I never delude myself that I can take the place of a veterinarian. When something beyond my competence comes up, I do what you should do—call the veterinarian.

APPENDIX A

Remedies and their Abbreviations

REMEDY	ABBREVIATED NAME	ABBREVIATIONS
Aconitum napellus	Aconite	Acon.
Aesculus hippocastanum	Aesculus	Aesc.
Allium cepa		All.c.
Alumina		Alum.
Anacardium		Anac.
Apis mellifica	Apis	Apis.
Antimonium crudum	Antimonium crud.	Ant.c.
Antimonium tartaricum	Antimonium tart.	Ant.t.
Arnica montana	Arnica	Arn.
Arsenicum album	Arsenicum	Ars.
Baryta carbonica	Baryta carb.	Bar.c.
Belladonna		Bell.
Berberis vulgaris	Berberis	Berb.
Bryonia alba	Bryonia	Bry.
Calcarea carbonica	Calcarea carb.	Calc.
Calcarea phosphorica	Calcarea phos.	Calc.p.
Calendula officinalis	Calendula	Calen.
Cantharis		Canth.
Carbolicum acidum	Carbolic acid	Carb.ac.
Carbo vegetabilis	Carbo veg.	Carb.v.
Caulophyllum		Caul.
Causticum		Caust.
Chamomilla		Cham.
Cinchona officinalis	China	Chin.
Cistus canadensis	Cistus	Cist.
Cocculus		Cocc.
Coffea cruda	Coffea	Coff.
Colchicum		Colch.
Collinsonia		Coll.
Colocynthis	Colocynth	Coloc.
Crotalus horridus	Crotalus	Crot.h.
Cuprum arsenicosum	Cuprum ars.	Cupr.ar.
Cuprum metallicum	Cuprum	Cupr.
Dulcamara		Dulc.
Echinacea augustifolia	Echinacea	Echi.
Equisetum		Equis.

REMEDY	ABBREVIATED NAME	ABBREVIATION
Eupatorium perfoliatum	Eupatorium	Eup.per.
Euphrasia		Euphr.
Ferrum metallicum	Ferrum met..	Ferr.m.
Ferrum phosphoricum	Ferrum phos.	Ferr.p.
Gelsemium sempervirens	Gelsemium	Gels.
Glonoine		Glon.
Graphites		Graph.
Hamamelis virginica	Hamamelis	Ham.
Hepar sulphuris calcareum	Hepar sulph.	Hep.
Hypericum perfoliatum	Hypericum	Hyper.
Ignatia amara	Ignatia	Ign.
Ipecacuanha	Ipecac.	Ip.
Kali bichromicum	Kali bi.	Kali.bi.
Kali bromatum	Kali brom.	Kali.br.
Kali carbonicum	Kali carb.	Kali.c.
Kali muriaticum	Kali mur.	Kali.m.
Kreosotum	Kreos.	Kreos.
Ledum palustre	Ledum	Led.
Lycopodium		Lyc.
Magnesia phosphorica	Magnesium phos.	Mag.p.
Mercurius corrosivus	Mercurius corr.	Merc.c.
Mercurius vivus	Mercurius	Merc.
Natrum muriaticum	Natrum mur.	Nat.m.
Natrum phosphoricum	Natrum phos.	Nat.p.
Nitricum acidum	Nitric acid	Nit.ac.
Nux vomica	Nux	Nux.v.
Oxalicum acidum	Oxalic acid	Ox.ac.
Phosphorus		Phos.
Phytolacca decandra	Phytolacca	Phyt.
Podophyllum		Podo.
Pulsatilla nigricans	Pulsatilla	Puls.
Pyrogenium	Pyrogen.	Pyrog.
Rhododendron		Rhod.
Rhus toxicodendron	Rhus tox.	Rhus.t.
Rumex crispus	Rumex	Rumx.
Ruta graveolens	Ruta	Ruta
Sabina		Sabin.
Sanguinaria		Sang.
Sepia		Sep.
Silicea or Silica		Sil.
Spongia tosta	Spongia	Spong.
Sulphur		Sulph.
Symphytum officinale	Symphytum	Symph.
Thuja occidentalis	Thuja	Thuj.
Urtica urens	Urtica	Urt.u.
Veratrum album	Veratrum alb.	Verat.a.
Verbascum		Verb.

APPENDIX B

Mini-Repertory

This Mini-Repertory, based on Dr. James Tyler Kent's *Repertory to the Homeopathic Materia Medica*, provides a guide to the principal symptoms of the twenty-eight remedies contained in the Home Remedy Kit. It will enable you to find the remedy most similar to the patient's symptoms in a reasonable amount of time. To use the Mini-Repertory:

1. Carefully observe your patient and note significant symptoms according to the Observation Checklist in chapter 3.
2. Look up each symptom in the Mini-Repertory to determine which remedy (or remedies) most strongly and consistently shows this symptom. When a remedy following a particular symptom is in all capital letters, this is the remedy of choice for that symptom.
3. To help you choose between two or more possible remedies, look up each remedy in the *Materia Medica* (Appendix C). This will lead you to the remedy that most closely fits the symptom picture of the patient.

We have omitted certain less frequently indicated remedies in an effort to simplify your task. Some of these other remedies may be indicated at times. If you don't find your symptoms or your remedies here, check the end-of-chapter summaries, which list the symptoms for specific ailments, and then use the *Materia Medica*.

A homeopathic physician may also choose one of those remedies not shown on your Mini-Repertory. In this case, the physician may be using a more complete repertory.

HOME REMEDY KIT : REPERTORY

OBSERVE :

1. Color.
    a. Skin
        Pale: Acon., ANT.T., Apis, Arn., ARS., Bell., Bry., CALC.P., Canth., CARBO V., Cham., FERR.P., Ign., Ip., Led., Mag.p. Merc., Nux v., Phos., Puls., Spong., SULPH., VERAT.
        Red: ACON., Ant.t., APIS, Arn., Ars., BELL., BRY., Canth., CHAM., Ferr.p., Hep., Hyper., Ign., Merc., NUX V., PHOS., Puls., Spong., Sulph., Verat.
        Circumscribed red: Ant.t., Ars., Ferr.p., PHOS., Puls., SULPH.
    b. Lips.
        Dry: Acon., Ant.t., Apis, Bell., BRY., Canth., Gels., Ign., Merc., Nux v., Phos., PULS., SULPH., Verat.a.
        Cracked: Arn,, Ars., BRY., CARBO V., Cham., Ign., Merc., Phos., SULPH., Verat.a.
        Red: Apis, ARS., Ferr.p., Puls.
        Pale: Apis, ARS., Ferr.p., Puls.

c. *Tongue*
   Dry: ACON., Ant., APIS, Arn., ARS., BELL., BRY., Calc.p., Carbo v., CHAM., Ip., MERC., Nux v., Phos., PULS., Spong., SULPH., Verat.a.
   Wet: Bell., Calc.p., Canth.; Carbo v., Cham., Ferr.p., Hep., Ign., IP., MERC., NUX V., Phos., Puls., Sulph., VERAT.A.
   Red: Acon., APIS, ARS., BELL., Canth., Carbo v., Cham., Ferr.p., Gels., MERC., Nux v., PHOS., Sulph., Verat.a.
   Red tip: Apis, ARS., SULPH.
   Red-streaked: Ant.t.
   White: Acon., Ant.t., Apis, Arn., ARS., BELL., BRY., Carbo v., Cham., Gels., Hyper., MERC., Nux v., Phos., PULS., SULPH.
   Swollen: ACON., APIS, Ars., BELL., Calc.p., Canth., MERC., Phos.

2. Expression
   a. *Anxious:* ACON., Ant.t., Apis, ARS., Bell., Carbo v., Nux v., Spong., Sulph., VERAT.A.,
   b. *Frightened:* ACON., Canth,
   c. *Stupefied:* Arn., Ars., Gels.
   d. *Confused:* Ars., Phos.
   e. *Drooping eyelids:* Ars., GELS.

3. Position and movement
   a. *Quite, still:* BRY., GELS.
   b. *Restless:* ACON., Apis, Ant.t., ARS., BELL., CALC.P., Carbo v., Cham., Led., MERC., Nux v., PULS., SULPH.
   c. *Lethargic:* BRY., GELS.

4. Mood
   a. *Irritable::* ACON., Ant.t,, APIS, Ars., BELL., BRY., Calc. p., Canth., CARBO V., CHAM., Gels., HEP., Led., Merc., NUX V., PHOS., PULS., Ruta, Spong., SULPH., Verat.a.
   b. *Nervous:* ACON., Ars., Bell., Bry., Cham., Ferr. p., Merc., NUX V., Phos., Puls.
   c. *Withdrawn:* GELS., Merc., PHOS., PULS., SULPH.
   d. *Angry:* ACON., Apis, ARS., Bell., BRY., Calc.p., Carbo v., CHAM., HEP,, IGN., Led., NUX V., Phos., SULPH.
   e. *Sad:* ACON., ARS., Bell., BRY., Calc.p., Canth., Carbo v., CHAM., Ferr.p,, GELS., Hep., IGN., Ip., MERC., Nux v., Phos., PULS., Ruta, Spong., SULPH., VERAT.A.

FEEL :

1. Skin
   a. *Dry:* Acon., Ant.t., Apis, Arn., ARS., BELL., BRY., Carbo v., CHAM., Ip., LED., Merc., PHOS., Puls., Spong., SULPH., Verat a.
   b. *Moist:* Ant.t., ARS., CARBO V., HEP., Led., MERC., Phos., Puls., Spong., Sulph.
   c. *Hot:* ACON., APIS, ARS., BELL., BRY., Hep., Ign., Merc., Nux v., PHOS., Puls., SULPH.
   d. *Cool or cold:* Ant.t., ARS., Bell., CALC.P., Carbo v., Cham., Ign., IP., Led., Merc., Nux v., Phos., SULPH., VERAT.A.
   e. *Sensitive:* Acon., APIS, BELL., Bry., Ferr.p., HEP., Ip., Led., Nux v., MERC., SULPH.
   f. *Clammy:* Ant.t , Carbo v., Verat.a.

2. Pulse
   a. *Rapid:* ACON., Ant.t., APIS, ARN., ARS., BELL., BRY., Canth., Cham., FERR.P., GELS., Hyper., Ign., MERC., NUX V., PHOS., Puls., Spong., SULPH., Verat.a.
   b. *Slow:* Acon., Ant.t., Bell., Canth., GELS., Verat.a.
   c. *Weak:* ANT.T., Arn., ARS., Canth., CBRBO V., GELS., Ign., Ip., Merc., Phos., Puls.
   d. *Hard:* ACON., Ant.,t. Arn., BELL., BRY., Canth., Hep., Ign., Led., Merc., Nux v., Phos., Sulph.

3. Response to Touch
   a. *Pain:* Acon., Ant.t., APIS, ARN., Ars., BELL., BRY., Canth., Carbo v., CHAM., HEP., Led., MAG.P., Merc., NUX V., Phos., Puls., Spong., SULPH., Verat.a.
   b. *Withdrawal:* Acon., Ant.t., Arn., Bell., Bry., CHAM.
   c. *Comforted:* Ars., Bry., Phos.

LISTEN :

1. Voice
   a. *Weak:* Ant.t., Bell., CANTH., Carbo v., Cham., Ferr.p., Gels., HEP., Ign., Nux v., Phos., Puls., Spong., Sulph., VERAT.A,
   b. *Hoarse:* ACON., ALL.C., Ant.t., Apis, Ars., BELL., BRY., Calc.p., Canth., CARBO V., CHAM., Gels., HEP., MERC., PHOS., Puls., SPONG., Sulph., Verat.a.
   c. *Deep:* CARBO V., Phos.
   d. *Husky:* Acon., PHOS., Spong., Sulph.
2. Breathing
   a. *Gasping:* Acon., Ant.t,, APIS, Ars., Hyper., Ip., Phos., Spong.
   b. *Rapid:* ACON., ANT.T., Arn., ARS., BELL., BRY., Canth., CARBO V., Cham., GELS., Hep., Ign., IP., Merc., Nux v., PHOS., Puls., SULPH., Verat.a.
   c. *Difficult:* Acon., ANT.T., APIS., Arn., ARS., Bell., BRY., CARBO V., Ferr.p., Gels., HEP., Ign., IP., Merc., Nux v., PHOS., PULS., SPONG., SULPH., VERAT.A.
   d. *Wheezing:* ARS., CARBO V., Cham., IP.
   e. *Irregular:* Ant.t., Ars., BELL., Cham., Ign., Nux v., Puls.
3. Speech
   a. *Incoherent:* Bell., BRY., Gels., PHOS., Sulph.
   b. *Hasty:* Bell., HEP., Ign., MERC.
   c. *Slow:* Phos.
   d. *Refuses to answer:* Arn., Nux v., PHOS., SULPH., Verat.a.
4. State of Mind
   a. *Irrational:* Acon., Ars., Bell., IGN., SULPH.
   b. *Delirious:* Acon., ARS., BELL., BRY., Cham. Gels., Ip., Merc., Nux v., Phos., Puls., Sulph., VERAT.A.
5. Complaints
   a. Location
   Head: ACON., APIS, Arn., ARS., BELL., BRY., Cham., Ferr.p., GELS., Hep.s., Ign., Ipec., Led., MAG.P., Merc., NUX V., PHOS., PULS., Ruta, SULPH.
   Eye: Acon., All.c., Apis, Arn., Ars., BELL., BRY., Calc.p., CHAM., Ferr.p., Gels., Hep., Ign., Mag.p., MERC., Nux v., Phos., Puls., RUTA, Spong., Sulph.
   Ear: Acon., All.c., Apis, Arn., Ars., BELL., Calc.p., Carbo.v., CHAM., Gels., HEP., Mag.p., MERC., Nux v., PHOS., PULS., Spong., SULPH.
   Nose: Ars., HEP., Merc., PULS., Sulph.
   Teeth: ACON, Ars., BELL., BRY., Carbo v., CHAM., HEP., MERC., Nux v., Phos., Puls., Sulph.
   Throat: Apis, BELL., Hep., Ign., Merc., Phos., Sulph.
   Stomach: Acon., Ant.t., Apis, Arn., ARS., BELL., BRY., Calc.p., Canth., CARBO V., Cham., Gels., Ign., Ip, Mag.p., Merc., NUX V., PHOS., PULS., SULPH., VERAT.A.
   Chest: Acon., ARN., APIS, ARS., BELL, BRY., CALC.P., Canth., Carbo v., Cham., Hep., Mag.p., Merc., Nux v., PHOS., Puls., SPONGIA., Sulph., Verat.
   Abdomen: All.c., Apis, ARS., Bell., BRY., Calc.p., CANTH., Carbo v., CHAM., IP., Led., Nux v., PHOS., PULS., Sulph., VERAT.
   Rectum: Acon., Ars., Bell., Carbo v., IGN., Merc., Nux v., Phos., PULS., Ruta, SULPH.
   Bladder: Acon., Apis, Ars., BELL., Calc.c., CANTH., Carbo v., Puls.

Uterus: Acon., BELL., Bry., Calc.p., Cham., Gels., NUX V., PULS.
Ovaries: Acon., APIS, BELL., Bry., Ign., MAG.P., Merc., Phos., Puls.
Vagina: Bell, Calc.p., Cham., Merc., Nux v., Puls., Sulph.
Neck: Acon., Apis, ARS., BELL., Bry., Calc.p. Carbo v., Ferr.p., GELS., Hep., Ign., Ip., Mag.p., Merc., Phos., Puls.
Upper back: Bell., Bry., Calc.p., Hyper., Merc., Phos., SULPH.
Lower back: Apis, Arn., BRY., Calc.p., CANTH., Carbo v., Cham., Ferr.p., Gels., Hep., Ip., LED., Mag.p., NUX V., PHOS., PULS., Ruta, SULPH.
Sacroiliac region: Ant.t., Bry., Calc.p.
Hips: Acon., Arn., ARS., Bell., Bry., Calc.p., HEP., LED., Merc., Phos., PULS., Sulph., Verat.a.
Thigh: Apis, Ars., Bell., Bry., Carbo v., Gels., Hep., Hyper., Led., Merc., Sulph.
Legs: Arn., Ars., BELL., Gels., Led., Merc., Nux v., Phos., Puls., Sulph., Verat.a.
Feet: Apis, Arn., Ars., Carbo v., Led., Merc., Nux v., Ruta, Verat.a.
Shoulders: Ars., Bry., Calc.p., Ferr.p., Hep., Ign., Led., Merc., Phos., Puls., SULPH.
Arms: Ars., BRY., Calc.p., Cham., Gels., Hep., Led., Mag.p., Nux v., Phos., PULS., Sulph., Verat.a.
Hands: Hep., Sulph.
Fingers: Acon., Hep.

b. Time
Worse
Morning: Acon., Apis, Arn., Ars., BRY., CALC.P., CARBO V., CHAM., Ferr.p., Gels., Hep., Ign., Merc., NUX V., PHOS., PULS., SULPH., VERAT.A.
Noon: Apis, Ars., Carbo v., Phos., Sulph.
Afternoon: Apis, Ars., BELL., Bry., Calc.p., Canth., Ign., Led., Merc., Nux v., Phos., PULS., Sulph.
Evening: Acon., All.c., ANT.T., ARN., Ars., BELL., BRY., CARBO V., CHAM., Ferr.p. Hep., Ign., Ip., Led., MERC., Nux v., PHOS., PULS., RUTA, Spong., SULPH.,
Night: ACON., Ant.t., ARN., ARS., Bell., Bry., CALC.P., Canth., Carbo v., CHAM., Ferr.p., HEP., Ign., IP., Led., MERC., Nux v., PHOS., PULS., Spong., SULPH.

c. Kind of pain
Aching: Acon., Arn., Ars., Bell., Bry., Calc.p., Carbo v., Cham., Ip., Gels., Nux v., Phos., Puls., Sulph.
Boring: BELL., Hep., Merc., PULS., Sulph.
Bruised (sore): Acon., ARN., Bry., Canth., Led., Phos., Puls., RUTA.
Burning: Acon., APIS, Arn., ARS., Bell., BRY., Calc.p., CANTH, CARBO V., MERC., NUX V., PHOS., Puls., Spong., SULPH.
Bursting: Acon., BELL., BRY., Hep., Ip., MERC., PHOS., Puls., Spong., Sulph.
Cramping: Acon., Ant.t., Apis, Ars., BELL., Bry., Calc.p., CARBO V., Cham., Gels., Hep., IGN., IP., Led., MAG.P., Merc., NUX V., PULS., SPONG., SULPH., VERAT.A.
Cutting: ACON., Ant.t., Apis, ARS., Bry., CANTH., Cham., Hep., Ign., IP., Led., Merc., NUX V., Phos., PULS., SULPH., VERAT.A.
Dull: All.c., Apis, Gels., Hyper., Merc., NUX V., PULS.
Nail, as from: Hep., Ign., Nux v., Puls.
Pressing: Acon., Ant.t., Arn., Ars., Bell., Bry., Canth., Carbo v., Cham., Gels., Ign., Ip., Led., Merc., NUX V., PHOS., PULS., RUTA, Spong., SULPH., Verat.a.
Stitching: Acon., Arn., Ars., BELL., BRY., Calc.p., Canth., Gels., Ign., LED., MERC., Nux v., Phos., PULS., Spong., Sulph.

6. Desires
   a. Air
      Open: Apis, Arn., Ars., Bry., CARBO V., PULS., SULPH.
      With fanning: CARBO V.
   b. Food, cold: Ant.t., PHOS., PULS., Verat.a.

MINI-REPERTORY

 c. Drinks
  Cold: ACON., Ant.t., ARS., Bell., BRY., CHAM., Led., MERC., PHOS., VERAT.
  Warm: ARS., BRY., Carbo v., Hyper., Sulph.
 d. Cold applications: Led.
  Warm applications: ARS., MAG.P.
 e. Warmth in general: Acon., ARS., Bell., Bry., CALC.P., Carbo v., Cham., GELS., Hep., HYPER., Ign., IP., Led., LYC., MAG.P., Merc., NUX V., PHOS., Puls., Sulph.
 f. Cold in general: All.c., Ant.t., APIS., Bry., Ip., LED., Merc., Phos., PULS., Sulph., Verat.a.

SMELL :

1. Sick: All.c. ARN., ARS,, Bell., Bry., CARBO V., CHAM.. Gels., Hep., MERC., Puls., SULPH.
2. Sour: Acon., ANT.T., ARS., BELL., BRY., CARBO V., Ferr.p., Gels., HEP., Ip., MERC., Nux v., Phos., Puls., Spong., Sulph., VERAT.A.
3. Sweet: Apis, Merc., Puls.
4. Musty: Puls.
5. Offensive: ARN., Ars., Carbo v., HEP., MERC., NUX V., Phos., PULS., SULPH., Verat.a.

APPENDIX C
Materia Medica

ACONITUM NAPELLUS (ACONITE)

Ailments from fright; sudden onset and intense symptoms.
Anxiety and restlessness with any complaint.
Intolerant of pain, fears will not recover.
Pains followed by numbness and tingling.
Faintness or dizziness on rising.
Common cold, first stages only.
Fevers; sudden onset; hot, dry skin; often one cheek red, the other pale.
Thirst for large quantities of water, unquenchable.
Painful, red, hot, scanty urination, with anxiety.
Croup; when child wakens frightened from sleep with dry, hoarse, croupy cough. Usually the only remedy needed.
Eyes; relieves pain and aids healing in injuries such as a scratch on the eyeball, or pain from a foreign body in the eye.
Bursting, throbbing headache; sensation as if band around head.

WORSE FROM

evening and night
lying on affected side
warm room
music
tobacco smoke
dry, cold winds

BETTER FROM

open air

ALLIUM CEPA

Colds in damp, cold weather. Onset with sneezing. Streaming eyes and nose. Nasal discharge acrid, making upper lip and nose sore. Discharge from eyes is bland.
  Nose stuffed.
  Only one nostril dripping.
Hoarseness, beginning laryngitis.
Coughs from inhaling cold air. Grasps throat when coughing; feels as if cough would split or tear it.
Headache, mostly in forehead.
Neuralgic pains.
Indicated in colicky babies with pains in the abdomen.
Symptoms begin on the left side and extend toward the right.

MATERIA MEDICA

WORSE FROM	BETTER FROM
evening warm room	open air cold room

ANTIMONIUM TARTARICUM (ANTIMONIUM TART.)

Cough; rattling of mucus in chest, but nothing comes up.
Wheezing. Difficult breathing as if drowning in own secretions.
Face is cold, blue, pale, covered with cold sweat.
Great sleepiness.

WORSE FROM	BETTER FROM
damp, cold weather evening warmth all sour foods, milk	cold, open room sitting up belching spitting

APIS MELLIFICA (APIS)

Bee stings and insect bites with swelling, itching, and redness.
Hives.
Pains are stinging and burning.
Puffy swellings may be around the face, eyelids, eyes, mouth, or in throat.
Breathing difficult.
Thirstless.
Scanty urine.

WORSE FROM	BETTER FROM
heat touch bed is intolerable pressure right side late afternoon after sleeping closed, heated room	cold applications motion open air uncovering

ARNICA MONTANA (ARNICA)

Bruising injuries to soft tissues.
Injuries from blows, falls, or blunt objects.
Shock from injury.
Concussion of the brain.
Eye injuries, black eye.
Bleeding caused by injury.
Promotes healing.
Relieves soreness and bruised feeling following childbirth, illnesses, fractures, and surgery.
Soreness after tooth extraction or dental surgery.
Soreness of muscles from overexertion.

Sprains of joints, "tennis elbow."
Helpful even in old injuries.
Denies he or she is ill or that there is anything wrong,
Everything on which patient lies seems too hard.
Fear of being touched or of anyone's coming near.

WORSE FROM

light touch
heat
rest

BETTER FROM

lying down
with head low

ARSENICUM ALBUM (ARSENICUM)

Anxious, restless, fearful, irritable.
Weak and exhausted.
Desires air but is sensitive to the cold.
Later stages of head cold, with sneezing; red nose and eyes; and profuse, watery discharge.
Asthma worse after midnight; fears suffocation while lying down.
Burning pains, better from heat.
Sleepiness but unable to sleep; restlessness.
Thirsty for small drinks often.
Food poisoning.
Vomiting with or without offensive diarrhea after eating or drinking, followed by great weakness.

WORSE FROM

right side
after midnight
sight or smell of food
cold
cold drinks and food

BETTER FROM

warmth
head elevated
hot drinks

BELLADONNA

Restless, red, and hot.
Cold, flu, sore throat, cough, fever, headache, earache,
Earaches, especially the right ear, after getting the head cold or wet. Sudden onset.
Fever, especially in children. Pupils dilated, eyes bright.
Sudden and violent onset.
Skin dry and hot to the touch.
Eyes red, sensitive to the light, pupils dilated.
Throbbing, congestive headaches.
Sleepy but can't sleep. Restless sleep with muscular twitching.
Teething problems.
Sunstroke with pounding pulse.
Throbbing pains, worse from motion or jarring.
Vomiting from fright or nervousness.

WORSE FROM

motion
noise
jarring
light
lying down

BETTER FROM

standing or sitting erect

BRYONIA ALBA (BRYONIA)

Conditions with fever.
Dry, hard, spasmodic cough with stitches in the chest; must press hand to sternum. Cough worse at night, after eating and drinking, taking a deep breath, and when entering a warm room.
Headaches; head feels as if it would burst. Pain sharp from slightest cough. Thirsty, but drinking makes headache worse.
Wants to be quiet and left alone. Irritable. Wants things, which are refused when offered.
Pale.
Feverish.
Thirsty for large amounts of cold drinks at long intervals.
Constipated; stools large, dry, and hard.
Colic, vomiting from rich or fatty foods.
Rheumatism with red, swollen, hot, shiny joints. Motion, touch and pressure aggravate the pain.
Stitching pains, better from firm pressure, worse from motion.
Symptoms develop slowly, usually worse on right side.

WORSE FROM	BETTER FROM
motion	rest
light touch	firm pressure
warmth	lying on painful side, because it prevents motion
exertion	
eating	cold

CALCAREA PHOSPHORICA (CALC. PHOS.)

Pains in joints and bones, "growing pains."
Headaches of schoolchildren.
Delayed or difficult teething in children, rapid decay of teeth.
Delayed closure of fontanelles in top of child's head.
Debility with anemia, sweaty scalp.
Colic whenever child eats, feeble digestion.
Easy vomiting in children.
Craving for ham, bacon, smoked or salted meats.
Promotes milk flow for breastfeeding mothers, when other symptoms agree.
Fractures where bones do not unite or are slow to do so.
Sensations of numbness and crawling.

WORSE FROM	BETTER FROM
damp, cold, changeable weather	summer
mental exertion	warm, dry weather

CANTHARIS

Cystitis; frequent burning, painful urination.
Intolerable constant urge to urinate.
Burns and scalds with rawness and smarting, relieved by cold applications.
    Cantharis aids healing and takes away the burning sensation.
Burning sensation in esophagus and stomach.
Burning in soles of feet at night.
Unquenchable thirst with aversion to all fluids.
Bad effects of drinking coffee.

WORSE FROM	BETTER FROM
drinking coffee and cold water touch urinating	gentle massage

CARBO VEGETABILIS (CARBO VEG.)

Weakness; desire for fresh, cold air.
Sudden collapse from any cause.
Breath cold.
Limbs cold, bluish skin, sweat cold and clammy.
External or internal bleeding with steady oozing.
Internal burnings and external coldness.
Aversion to milk and meat.
All foods disagree, turn to gas, especially fats. Gas worse lying down.
Burning in the stomach with sour belching, flatulence, regurgitation of food, and heartburn.
Rattling cough with itching in the throat. Spasmodic cough with gagging, choking, and vomiting of mucus.
Hoarseness, worse evenings.
Has never fully recovered from the effects of some previous illness.

WORSE FROM	BETTER FROM
evenings warm, moist weather lying down fat foods wine coffee milk	fanning cold belching

CHAMOMILLA

Intolerance of pain; fainting and sweating from severe pain.
Sensitive, peevish, irritable children. Child asks for things, then flings them away; wants to be carried.
Painful teething with or without fever. Greenish diarrhea during teething.
Colic; painful, draws legs up.
One cheek hot, the other pale and cold.
Toothache better from cold. Worse from warm drinks and at night.
Earache with severe pain. Ears feel stopped.
Thirsty.

WORSE FROM	BETTER FROM
heat open air, wind night	being carried warm, wet weather

FERRUM PHOSPHORICUM (FERRUM PHOS.)

Early stages of all inflammatory problems, including head colds, earache, cough, pneumonia, bronchitis, pleurisy, and rheumatism.
Fever with gradual onset. Pale complexion with red cheeks. Soft and rapid pulse.

Hard, dry, tickling cough, with painful chest and hoarseness.
Throbbing headache that is better from cold applications.
Symptoms usually worse on right side.

WORSE FROM	BETTER FROM
at night	cold applications
motion	4 to 6 A. M.
	touch

GELSEMIUM SEMPERVIRENS (GELSEMIUM)

Summer colds with mild fever. Watery discharge from nose with much sneezing. Dry cough with sore throat.
Influenza.
Tiredness and aching of whole body. Limbs, head, eyelids feel heavy.
Chilled with chills up and down back.
Headache as if band around head. Scalp sore to the touch.
Sore throat with red tonsils. Difficult swallowing. Pain shoots from throat to ear.
Lack of thirst.
Dizziness, drowsiness, trembling, and dullness.
Bad effects of sun or hot weather.
Symptoms develop several days after exposure.
Nervousness, apprehension, anxiety prior to dental work or surgery.

WORSE FROM	BETTER FROM
damp weather	bending forward
emotion	open air
anticipation	continued motion
any effort to think	increased urination
thinking of one's ailments	stimulants
tobacco smoking	

HEPAR SULPHURIS CALCAREUM (HEPAR SULPH.)

Irritable. Chilly.
Great sensitivity mentally and physically.
Sensitive to cold, cold air, drafts. Feels as if wind is blowing on some part.
Faints from slight pain.
Cold sores, abscesses, boils, infected ears.
Cold begins with irritation in throat.
Sore, ulcerated nose. Sneezes when goes into cold, dry wind, nose runs; later there is a thick, offensive discharge.
Sore throat with splinter sensation. Pain extends to ears when swallowing.
Hoarseness with loss of voice.
Dry, hoarse cough. Worse whenever any part of body becomes uncovered.
Croup with loose, rattling cough.
This remedy also helps to localize infection.

WORSE FROM	BETTER FROM
dry, cold air	wet weather
touch	warmth
lying on painful side	wrapping head up
slightest draft	eating
cool air	

HYPERICUM PERFOLIATUM (HYPERICUM)

Helpful in injuries to nerves.
Puncture wounds from nails, bites, splinters.
Smashed fingertips, nails, or toes.
Pain shoots upward from the wound, especially up the limbs, or, in spinal injury, up and down the spine.
Severe concussions of the spine and the brain. Injury to the tailbone, or coccyx.
Bee stings, if pains shoot upward.
Dental surgery, including root canal work or tooth extraction.
Eye injury.
Relieves pain after operations.
Speeds healing of jagged cuts.
Painful burns, as a lotion: $\frac{1}{2}$ teaspoon to 1 cup water.

WORSE FROM	BETTER FROM
dampness	bending head back
fog	
touch	
cold	

IGNATIA AMARA (IGNATIA)

Emotional strain.
Mental stress.
Bad effects of grief, worry, shock, and disappointment.
Hysteria,
Sad, sighing, moody, changeable.
Hiccough and hysterical vomiting.
Insomnia.
Headache as if nail were driven out through the side. Often follows anger or grief. Worse from stooping.
Intolerance of tobacco.

WORSE FROM	BETTER FROM
morning	lying on the painful side
emotions	warmth
tobacco smoke	walking
coffee, brandy	hard pressure
strong odors	

IPECACUANHA (IPECAC.)

Persistent nausea and vomiting, with a clean tongue.
Nausea not relieved by vomiting.
Lack of thirst.
Asthma attacks.
Cough incessant and violent with every breath.
Nosebleed.
Gushing of bright, red blood.
Gasping for air.
Pale; cold sweat.
Pulse weak.

WORSE FROM

lying down
slightest motion
dry weather

LEDUM PALUSTRE (LEDUM)

Helpful for puncture wounds from sharp-pointed objects such as nails and splinters.
Insect stings, especially mosquitoes.
Animal bites and scratches.
Black eye caused by a blow.
Injured parts are cold and are relieved by cold applications.

WORSE FROM	**BETTER FROM**
warm applications	cold applications
heat of the bed	
night	

MAGNESIA PHOSPHORICA (MAGNESIUM PHOS.)

Intermittent, spasmodic pains and neuralgia.
Colic with gas, better from gentle pressure and warmth.
Colic with belching, which gives no relief.
Frequent hiccoughs with heartburn.
Cramping pains, in calves, writer's cramp, menstrual cramps if relieved by heat.
Toothache relieved by heat.
Symptoms usually worse on the right side.
General muscular weakness.

WORSE FROM	**BETTER FROM**
cold	warmth
touch	gentle pressure
night	bending double

MERCURIUS VIVUS (MERCURIUS)

Smarting, raw, sore throat. Tonsillitis.
Swollen, inflamed neck glands.
Abscessed ears, pus infection, boils.
Profuse sweating with no relief. Offensive odor.
Bad breath. Profuse, metallic-tasting saliva.
Very thirsty, even though mouth is moist.
Thick tongue with yellowish-whiter coating. Teeth leave an imprint on tongue.
Swollen gums with soreness about teeth.
Painful diarrhea with a "never get done" feeling.
Persistent urging to urinate with intensive burning.
Extremely sensitive to heat and cold.
Weak and trembling.

WORSE FROM	**BETTER FROM**
night	being at rest
warmth of bed	
during perspiration	
heat and cold	
damp weather	

NUX VOMICA (NUX)

Irritable, impatient, hypersensitive to noise, touch, light, odors, etc.
Nausea; vomiting; sour, bitter belching, especially after improper eating or overindulgence in food or drink. Worse in the morning and after eating.
Chilly, sensitive to drafts.
Bad effects of coffee, alcoholic beverages, tobacco, highly seasoned foods, loss of sleep, or strong drugs.
Constipation with frequent and ineffectual urging for stool.
Headache in back of head or over eyes, as if nail is driven in. Dizziness.
Colds from dry, cold weather.
Nose stuffed, especially at night and in the open air. Nose drips during the day and in a warm room.
Insomnia after mental strain, abuse of coffee, alcohol, tobacco. Wakens between 3 and 4 A.M., falls asleep at daybreak, unrefreshed on waking.

WORSE FROM	BETTER FROM
early morning	rest
mental exertion	evening
anger	strong pressure
eating	uninterrupted nap
dry weather	warmth
touch	
spices	
stimulants, narcotics	
cold	
open air	

PHOSPHORUS

Anxious, fearful, weak.
Profuse bleeding anywhere. Nosebleed from vigorous nose blowing. Bleeding gums.
Hoarseness, loss of voice.
Painful laryngitis; tight, heavy chest.
Croupy, dry, rasping, tickling, tight cough, which is very exhausting. Worse from talking or breathing cold air.
Burning pains in stomach, intestines, and between shoulder blades.
Thirst for ice-cold drinks, which are vomited as soon as they become warm in the stomach.
Nausea.
Symptoms are worse on the left side.
Appears to be well despite high temperature.
Sweats at night.

WORSE FROM	BETTER FROM
evening	open air
lying on left or painful side	sleep
physical or mental exertion	rubbing
thunderstorms	cold food or drink
change of weather	
getting wet in hot weather	
warm food or drink	
touch	

PULSATILLA NIGRICANS (PULSATILLA)

Sensitive, weepy; desires attention and sympathy.
Changeable symptoms.
Craves open air; sensitive to heat.
Dryness of mouth with lack of thirst.
Stomach upsets from rich foods. Aversion to fats.
Fainting from hot stuffy atmosphere.
Insomnia from recurring thought.
"Ripe" head colds with profuse, thick, yellowish discharge. Eyelids stick together in the morning. Styes.
Loose, rattling cough; worse on becoming heated and at night.
Earache with thick yellow discharge. External ear swollen and red.
Often indicated in allergies, as hayfever, asthma, eczema.
Helpful in childhood diseases such as measles, mumps, and chickenpox.
To dry up mother's milk when no longer needed.
Delayed menstrual period with painful, scanty flow.

WORSE FROM

twilight
rich, fatty food
after eating
warm room
lying on left or painless side

BETTER FROM

motion
open air
cold food and drinks, though not thirsty
cold applications

RUTA GRAVEOLENS (RUTA)

Sprains (after *Arnica*), especially of tendons.
Helps in sprains of knees, wrists, ankles.
Injured, "bruised" bones, eyes, rectum, periosteum (the membrane surrounding the bone).
Painful, bruised skin.
Sciatica; worse lying down at night.
Red, hot eyes. Eyestrain followed by headache.
Deep aching.
"Dry socket" following dental extraction.

WORSE FROM

being at rest
lying down
cold, wet weather
cold

SPONGIA TOSTA (SPONGIA)

Croup, colds, and coughs beginning in the throat, which is sensitive to touch. Feeling as if there's a plug in the larynx.
Wakes fearfully out of sleep with a sense of suffocation, loud cough, difficult breathing.
Croupy cough, sounds like a saw driven through a board. Dry, barking, rasping cough.
Dryness of all air passages.
Hoarseness with soreness and burning.
Exhaustion and heaviness of the body after slight exertion.
Symptoms are similar to *Hepar sulph.* symptoms except that the *Spongia* patient is warm while the *Hepar sulph.* patient is chilly.

WORSE FROM	BETTER FROM
before midnight	lying with head low
lying down	
talking	
swallowing	
waking	

SULPHUR

Dry, scaly, unhealthy skin, with itching and burning; offensive odor. Worse from scratching and washing.
Red orifices: lips, eyelids, anus.
Burning heat: of palms of hands, top of head, and especially soles of feet; at night, uncovers feet, throws off bedcovers.
Uncomfortable when standing.
Dislike of water. Bathing makes patient feel worse.
Hypoglycemic symptoms: sinking feeling in stomach an hour before lunch time.
Thirsty; would rather drink than eat.
Bitter taste in the morning.
Painless diarrhea drives patient out of bed in early morning.
Constipation with hard, dry, large stools; held back because of pain; helpful in anal fissures (cracks inside anus); burning.
Sometimes helpful in failure to recover completely from acute ailments; as when colds, coughs, influenzas hang on too long.

WORSE FROM	BETTER FROM
morning	dry, warm weather
night	lying on right side
washing	
sleeping	
rest	
standing	
warmth of bed	
time to time	
alcoholic stimulants	

VERATRUM ALBUM (VERATRUM ALB.)

Nausea with violent vomiting and profuse diarrhea, clammy sweating and collapse.
Cramping, watery diarrhea.
Heat exhaustion.
Sudden collapse with coldness, blueness, and weakness.
Clammy sweat. Cold sweat on forehead.
Pulse rapid and weak.
Cramps in abdomen, legs, and calves.

WORSE FROM	BETTER FROM
night	warmth
least motion	walking
drinking	
during stool	
after fright	

APPENDIX D

Consumer's Guide to Homeopathic Medicine

IN homeopathy, the quality of medicine is of paramount importance in comparison to other systems of treatment. This is so because in this system only the essence or the inherent power of the drug called "potency" is used to cure diseases.

Drugs are available in various forms, such as, mother tinctures, globules, pillules, sugar of milk, etc. These can be bought from any reputable homeopathic drug store. These are prepared in India as well as imported from abroad.

Drugs made in foreign countries are regarded as better and the best are from Boericke & Tafel (popularly known as B & T), U.S.A. The second best are from Germany, namely, Madaus & Co., and William Schwabe.

In India, Calcutta is the birthplace of homeopathy. There are several drug manufacturing companies, the best being Hahnemann Publishing Co., popularly known as HAPCO. Other Calcutta-based companies are: (1) National Homeopathic Laboratory, (2) Economic Homeo Laboratory, (3) Hahnemann Laboratory (not the one mentioned above), etc. Certain other well-known companies are: Ramakrishna Pharmaceuticals, Hyderabad; Sri Krishna Homeo Pharmacy, Pune; Hahnemann Scientific Laboratory, Lucknow; St. George Homeo Pharmacy, Mangalore; Bhandari Homeopathic Laboratory, Faridabad (near Delhi); Wheezal Laboratories, Dehradun; etc.

The American and German medicines are relatively costlier. If one wants to buy these for better results, he should insist on sealed packings. Even otherwise the buyer should check the name of the company.

Wooden boxes in various sizes, even in pocket size, are available at drug stores. One can buy these for preparing his own Medical Kit.

—DR. R.S. BANSAL

Also in Orient Paperbacks

The Complete Book of HOME REMEDIES

Hakeem H. Abdul Hameed Saheb
Hamdard Dawakhana and Laboratories

pp 158
Rs. 50.00

This book is a detailed authoritative health home-reference manual on all aspects of home medical-care. There are separate chapters covering over 130 minor and major ailments and disorders—including fevers, headaches, throat problems, digestive disorders, problems of the eyes, ears and nose, diarrhoea, diabetes, blood-pressure, colic pain, haemorrhoids, obesity, nausea and much more—their causes, symptoms and specific home-remedies. There is a separate section on commonly available natural herbs, substances and minerals, their health-usefulness and curative properties.

"An authoritative manual for home reference... outlines simple practical remedies as well as preventive measures... invaluable for every family."

Times of India

"Home health care manual that helps to control and cure a variety of minor and major ailments."

Indian Express

"Hameed has done a thorough job and has systematically listed various kinds of maladies, their symptoms, and their detailed remedies."

Illustrated Weekly

"The author has attempted to appraise the common man of the value of home remedies. He has systematically dealt with diseases of the various organs and systems of the body, their signs and symptoms, remedies and regimen."

Tribune

"The author points out that home remedies have a tremendous scope and offer the only hope in terms of cheapness as well as access."

Femina

Available at all bookshops or by VPP

ORIENT PAPERBACKS
**Madarsa Road, Kashmere Gate
Delhi-110 006**